what you should know

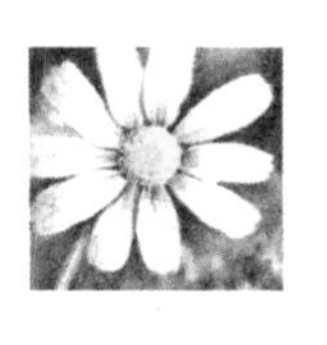

Women's Health Under 40

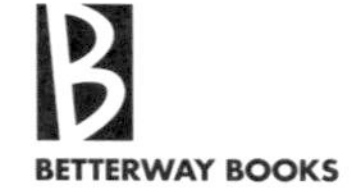

BETTERWAY BOOKS

what you should know

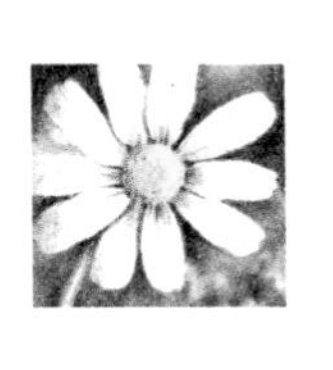

Women's Health Under 40

Written by Caroline J. Böhme, MD,
and Rona B. Wharton, MEd, RD, LD
Illustrated by Laura L. Seeley

First Edition.

Written by: Caroline J. Böhme, MD, and Rona B. Wharton, MEd, RD, LD
Contributing Editors: Douglas Wetherill, MS Dean J. Kereiakes, MD, FACC
Paul Ribisl, PhD
Illustrated by: Laura L. Seeley

Women's Health Under 40: What You Should Know™ is a trademark of Robertson & Fisher Publishing Company. Published by Betterway Books, an imprint of F&W Publications, Inc., 1507 Dana Avenue, Cincinnati, Ohio 45207.

A catalog record for this book is available from the U.S. Library of Congress.

Printed in Canada

This book is dedicated ...

To my husband Eric, to my family and all of my friends. — Caroline

To Sian & Megan, Katie & Lindsey — may you have long and happy lives! — Rona

To the memory of Mary Smalley and Mary Hill Moffit Linder who helped inspire this series. Thankfully, their wisdom, humor, and zest for life lives on through their children: Janet, Robert, Mary Brooks, Ralph, Cathy, Bobbie, and Anne.

To the memory of Mary A. Conlon. Mary's ability to give was surpassed only by her capacity to love others.

The authors are grateful to the following individuals for their input: Peggy Marquette, Janette Weisbrodt, Lynne Haag, Dr. Jennifer Thie, Dr. Andrew Botschner, Melissa Kircher, Jennifer Wyder, Dorothy and Steven Stoller, Richard Hunt, Phil Sexton, Sara Dumford, and Cecily Auvil.

Treatment Disclaimer

This book is for education purposes, not for use in the treatment of medical conditions. It is based on skilled medical opinion as of the date of publication. However, medical science advances and changes rapidly. Furthermore, diagnosis and treatment are often complex and involve more than one disease process or medical issue to determine proper care. If you believe you may have a medical condition described in the book, consult your doctor.

Table of Contents

Introduction viii
Anatomy 1
Pap Smears and Cervical Cancer 10
Abnormal Periods 33
Painful Periods 50
Vaginal Infections 64
Sexually Transmitted Diseases 71
Birth Control 84
Breast Cancer 100
Staying Healthy 132
Exercise 150
Questions 172
Woman to Woman 177

Introduction

Women experience many changes, emotionally and physically, throughout life. We also face many health issues that can be complicated, confusing, and sometimes frightening. In writing this book, our goal is to explain some common health issues women age 40 and younger can experience and make them more understandable. We hope to make it easier for you to talk to your doctor about health concerns.

— Caroline and Rona

Anatomy

Pelvic anatomy

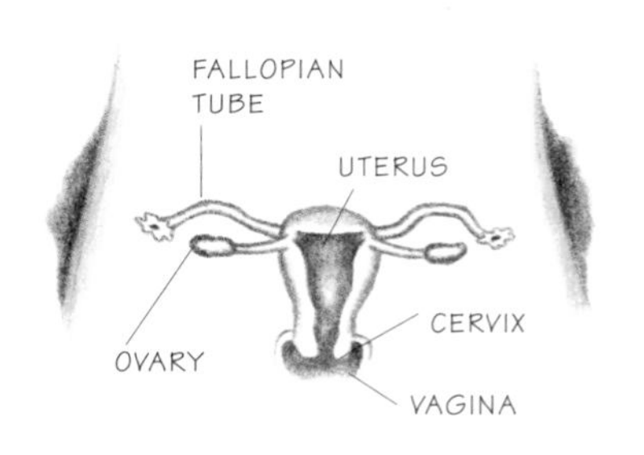

Understanding female anatomy is the first step to understanding what health issues specifically affect a woman. A woman has 2 **ovaries**, 2 **fallopian tubes**, a **uterus**, **cervix**, and **vagina**. The ovary is the storage house for eggs and plays a major role in the production of estrogen. The fallopian tubes are important for the transportation of eggs.

The uterus has a lining known as the **endometrium**. This lining sheds every month when a woman has a period. It also becomes the womb for pregnancy. The uterus is composed of smooth muscle known as the **myometrium**.

The cervix is the opening to the uterus and is the connection to the vagina. The cervix has an external portion and an internal portion.

The outside anatomy of a woman's vagina is known as the **vulva**. The **labia** — both the **minora** and **majora** — surround the vaginal opening. The **urethra** is located above the vagina and is the opening where urine is released.

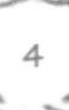

Anatomy of the breast

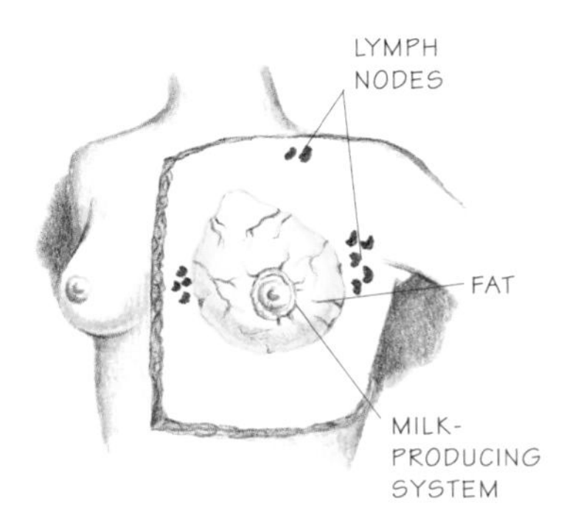

Women's ribs are covered with chest muscles. A lining covers these muscles. The breast itself is composed of **fat**, **lymph vessels**, **blood vessels**, and the **milk-producing system**. The lymph vessels lead to **lymph nodes** under the arm, above the collarbone, and in the chest. The lymph system is the "fighter" system in our bodies.

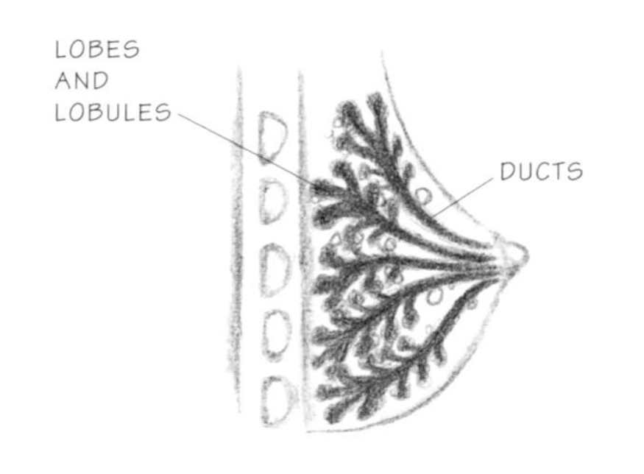

Each breast has about 20 sections that are called **lobes.** Each lobe ends in milk-producing glands or **lobules.** Thin tubes called **ducts** connect the lobules to the **nipple** to allow for the passage of milk.

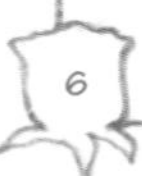

Menstruation

Menses begins when a female goes through puberty. The first menstrual period, known as **menarche**, is a signal that a woman's body is beginning to release eggs. The onset of menses is controlled by many different hormones. When a woman releases an egg each month, it is known as **ovulation**. Ovulation occurs about 14 days prior to when the period begins. So, if a woman's menstrual cycle is 28 days long, ovulation generally occurs on day 14.

When a woman ovulates and the egg does not get fertilized, she has a period. During a period, the lining of the uterus, which thickens in preparation for pregnancy, is shed.

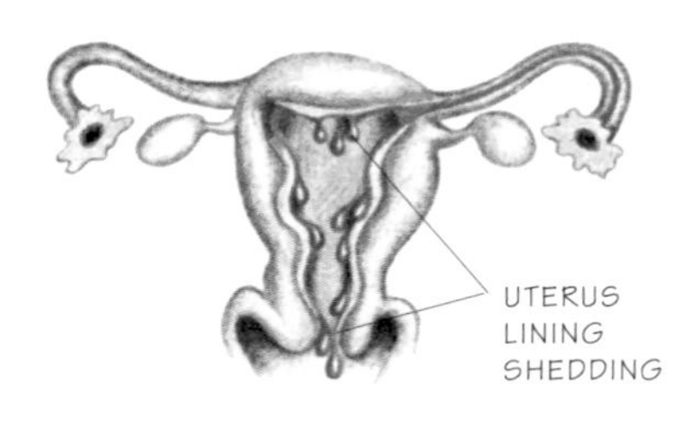

When a female is born, she has 2 million eggs. By puberty, the number of eggs decreases to about 500,000. When a woman reaches menopause, the egg supply is depleted.

A female generally has a period and ovulates every month. Sometimes it can take 1 to 2 years for an adolescent female to develop regular menstrual cycles after menses begins.

Pap Smears and Cervical Cancer

Why do we need a yearly exam?

A woman needs to see her doctor annually for a pelvic examination once she is sexually active or when she turns 18. It is important to have a pelvic examination to ensure that the female organs, both internal and external, are normal. It is also important to get a Pap smear every year. This may vary depending on your sexual practices, history of results of Pap smears, and whether or not you have

a cervix. It will be up to your doctor to decide how often you need a Pap smear. A breast exam is generally performed at the yearly exam as well.

Your doctor can answer any questions you may have about your health, including menstruation, pelvic discomfort, sexuality, birth control, and more.

What is a Pap smear and how is it performed?

The Pap smear was developed by Dr. George Papinicolou. It is a screening test for cervical cancer. Since its introduction, the test has decreased the incidence of cervical cancer by about 70%. It is one of the best screening tests available for the prevention of cancer.

A woman must have an internal exam to have a Pap smear. When a medical instrument known as a **speculum** is placed inside the vagina, it can be opened to allow your doctor to see your cervix. After inserting the speculum, your doctor gently removes **cells** from your cervix for evaluation. The cells are taken from inside and outside the cervix.

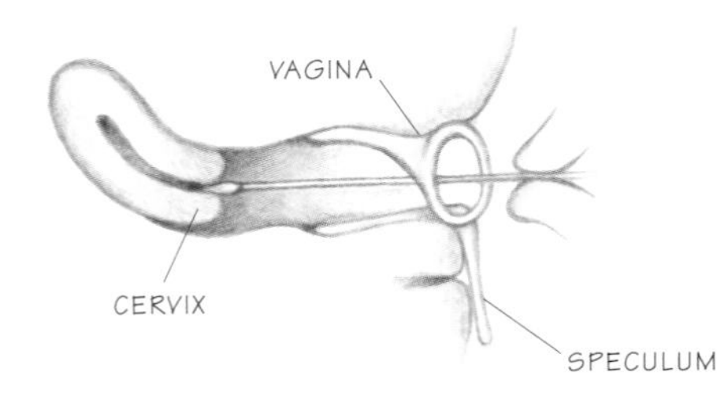

Your doctor also looks at your cervix and vagina for infection and other abnormalities. When a doctor performs a **speculum exam**, it does not necessarily mean that you will have a Pap smear. Check with your doctor to make sure you have had your Pap smear as often as your doctor recommends.

Abnormal Pap smears

The goal of a Pap smear is to detect **precancerous cells** early, before they develop into cervical cancer. Different stages of precancerous growth can occur and be treated. Generally, it takes years for Pap smear results to go from "normal" to cancer. There are instances when cancer can develop within a year, but these situations are rare.

The changes that can occur to the cells of the cervix are much like steps on a ladder. There are incremental, step-like changes of the cells going from normal to cancerous. Each rung of the ladder, as one goes higher, correlates with a more severe precancerous state.

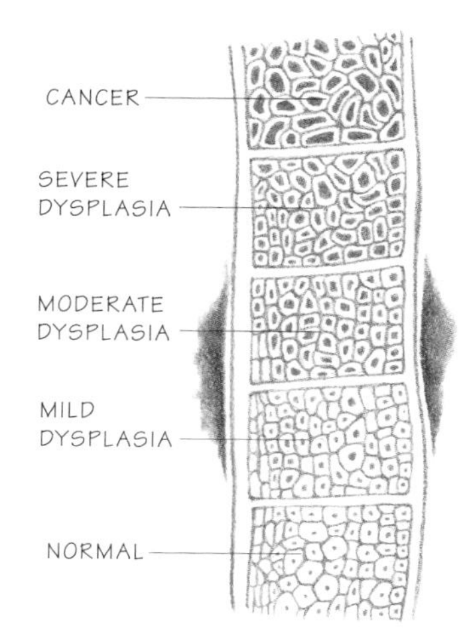

Many different terms are used to describe changes in the cells of the cervix. Pap smear results are categorized as follows:

- Normal
- Atypical
- Mild dysplasia
- Moderate dysplasia
- Severe dysplasia
- Cancer

Normal

When a woman has a normal Pap smear, she usually does not need a repeat Pap smear until 1 year later. Some doctors say that if a woman is monogamous and has had 3 normal Pap smears in a row, she may be able to have a Pap smear every 2 to 3 years. However, the general consensus is to continue with Pap smears every year.

Atypical

This is the next level or step of Pap smear result just after normal. A woman who has an atypical Pap smear needs to have the test repeated within 3 to 6 months. Some doctors may proceed with a test called a **colposcopy** after finding an atypical Pap smear. The majority of the atypical changes on a Pap smear may disappear on a follow-up Pap smear. Some doctors will perform a colposcopy after 2 consecutive atypical Pap smears.

There is also a Pap smear result known as an **atypical glandular Pap smear**. When your doctor finds this result, he or she may perform a colposcopy right away. You also may need a biopsy of your uterine lining known as an **endometrial biopsy**.

What is a colposcopy?

A colposcopy is performed by your doctor to take a closer evaluation of the cervix. A microscope is used to look at the cervix after the cervix is stained with acetic acid (which is basically vinegar). The vinegar solution stains abnormal cells white, enabling the doctor to evaluate them.

Other changes of the cervix, including blood vessel abnormalities, are evaluated. Your doctor will biopsy the cervix in the areas where abnormalities appear. The inside of the cervix is also sampled. The findings of the colposcopy will help your doctor determine the appropriate treatment.

Mild dysplasia

This is the next step beyond an atypical Pap smear. When a woman has this level of Pap smear result, she needs to have a follow-up colposcopy. A colposcopy is performed to make sure the cells of the cervix have not changed into a more severe precancerous state. Seventy percent of cases of mild dysplasia will disappear within a year.

Thirty percent of cases will stay the same or progress to a higher form of dysplasia.

If mild dysplasia persists for a year, some doctors advocate treatment, which involves removing the abnormal cells of the cervix. (We discuss treatment options on pages 29 to 32.)

Moderate dysplasia or severe dysplasia

When a woman has these findings on her Pap smear, she will need a colposcopy. Again, your doctor will want to make sure that the cells do not have more advanced changes. Most doctors will proceed with treatment of this condition after confirmation by the colposcopy results. Treatment for moderate or severe dysplasia also involves removing the specific abnormal cells of the cervix.

Cervical cancer

This finding requires aggressive treatment. There are different types of treatment depending on the stage of the cancer. Treatments include **surgery**, **radiation**, **chemotherapy**, or a combination of these. Your doctor can review this with you. You will need to see a gynecologic cancer specialist for treatment of cervical cancer.

Human papillomavirus (HPV)

This virus is transmitted through sexual intercourse. There are many different types of HPV. The reason it is important to know about HPV is that it is considered a possible cause of **dysplasia** of the cervix. Certain types appear to be associated with changing the cells of the cervix. The theory behind HPV is that it infects the cells of the cervix and causes abnormal cellular change. A few types of the virus are associated with **condyloma**, also known as **genital warts**.

Treatment

Different treatments are available for changes of cells in the cervix. Which treatment is right for you will depend on the type of cellular change, size, and extent of the lesion. The treatments we describe are for **precancerous changes.** Precancerous changes are not the same thing as cancer. If certain cellular changes are left untreated, they may develop into cancer.

There are 4 major treatments for changes in the cells of the cervix. Generally, most doctors do not treat changes of the cervix until the cells reach **mild dysplasia**. Even this state can be followed watchfully for a period of time, depending on the opinion of your doctor.

Treatment options

Cryotherapy

With cryotherapy, the abnormal cells of the cervix are frozen.

Laser treatment

Laser treatment burns up the abnormal cells of the cervix.

Loop Electrosurgical Excision Procedure (LEEP)

This procedure removes the abnormal cells of the cervix with a hot wire. The specimen removed can be sent to the lab for further evaluation to make sure all the abnormal cells have been removed. Also, the lab can make sure the cells are not more abnormal than originally diagnosed.

Cone biopsy

This is generally done in the operating room. The abnormal cells are removed with a surgical knife or scalpel. These cells can be sent to the lab for further evaluation. A cone biopsy may need to be performed if the colposcopy was inadequate or if there is a major discrepancy between the results of the colposcopy and the Pap smear.

Abnormal Periods

Abnormal periods

Many women suffer from irregularities in their menstrual cycles. A normal menstrual cycle can last from 21 to 35 days. Any differences in the timing of the menstrual cycle can be frustrating. Skipping periods or having too many bleeding episodes in a month can be either bothersome or worrisome. **Metrorrhagia** is the term used to describe a menstrual cycle occurring in irregular intervals with excessive flow and duration.

Some women suffer from increasingly heavy periods. This is known as **menorrhagia**.
If you suffer from changes in the timing or the heaviness of your period, you need to consult with your doctor to determine why this is occurring.

Physical reasons for changes in periods

Physical reasons for abnormal uterine bleeding include uterine fibroids, uterine polyps, and hyperplasia of the lining of the uterus. Pregnancy could also be a possibility. Cancer of the cervix and/or uterus also needs to be considered with abnormal bleeding, but these are rare conditions. Trauma to the genital organs and infection also may cause bleeding problems.

Uterine fibroids

Uterine fibroids are **benign** (noncancerous) muscle tumors of the uterus. By age 40, approximately 40% of women may have fibroids. Their presence can lead to painful periods, pelvic pressure, and abnormal uterine bleeding. Fibroids tend to cause heavier periods. Treatment for fibroids includes both medicinal and surgical methods. The medical treatment includes different hormonal regimens. (We further explore fibroids in the pelvic pain section, page 53).

Polyps

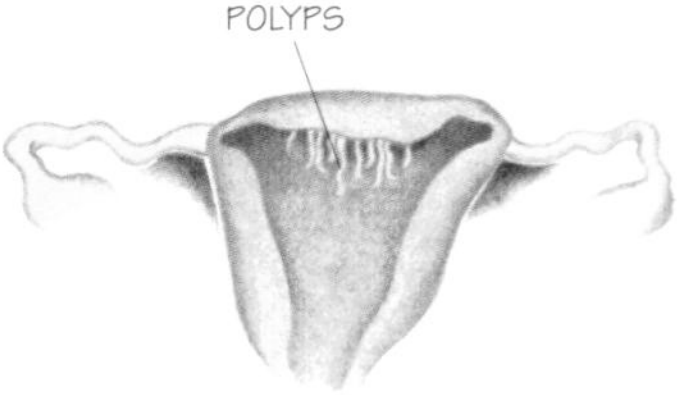

Uterine and cervical polyps can also cause irregular uterine bleeding. These can cause heavier periods or even spotting between periods. Polyps are finger-like projections of tissue that can be found along the uterine lining. They can also occur on or in the cervix. Generally, polyps need to be removed to resolve the bleeding problem. Polyps sometimes can be seen on a physical exam. They also can be diagnosed by an **endometrial biopsy**.

POLYPS

An endometrial biopsy allows your doctor to obtain a sample of the lining of the uterus. Polyps may also be evaluated with a **pelvic ultrasound**.

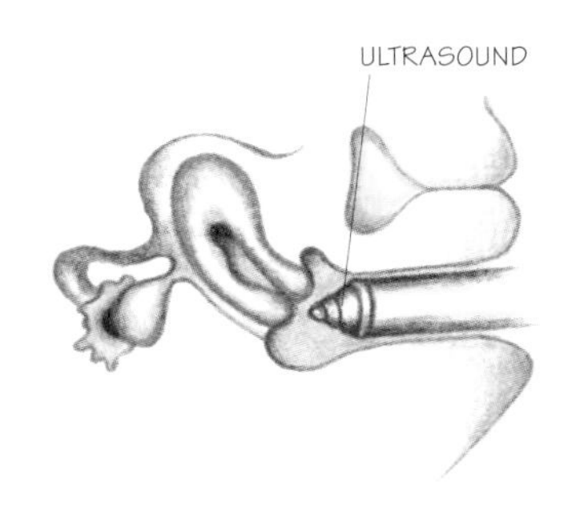

A pelvic ultrasound is performed to obtain a clearer view of the pelvic organs. The ultrasound probe is placed in a woman's vagina — close to the female internal organs. Sometimes a woman may need a full bladder prior to this procedure.

Hyperplasia

A thickening of the lining of the uterus, this condition can cause heavy periods or spotting between periods. Hyperplasia may be diagnosed with an endometrial biopsy. The treatment for hyperplasia is generally a hormone known as **progesterone**.

Sometimes abnormal cells can be found in the tissues. This is known as **atypical hyperplasia**. If a woman has atypical hyperplasia and wants to have children, she may be treated with high-dose progesterone therapy and a **D&C (dilatation and curettage)**. If a woman is not planning to become pregnant, then a hysterectomy may be the best option. Atypical cells found in the lining of the uterus may lead to cancer of the uterus if left untreated.

Hormonal and medical reasons for changes in periods

A lot of factors can change the normal menstrual cycle a woman experiences. If a woman does not ovulate regularly, this is known as **anovulation**. Anovulation may also lead to menstrual irregularities. Other life factors such as excessive weight gain or weight loss and extreme stress can also affect a woman's menstrual cycle and can possibly lead to bleeding abnormalities.

Thyroid disease is another problem that can lead to abnormal bleeding. The thyroid gland is located in the neck. If the thyroid is overactive, this is known as **hyperthyroidism**. If it is underactive, this is known as **hypothyroidism**. If either of these conditions is found, it needs to be corrected. This correction may lead to normalization of the menstrual cycle.

Some women who have bleeding disorders may have heavy, regular cycles from the onset of menses. These women may also have other bleeding tendencies including prolonged or frequent bleeding when brushing their teeth or when they cut themselves. Certain hormonal medications can cause bleeding problems. Blood thinner medication and some herbs may lead to bleeding abnormalities. If a woman does not have a physical reason for abnormal bleeding, her doctor must look for a hormonal or medical reason. If you are experiencing irregular cycles, spotting between periods, or having heavier periods than normal, contact your doctor right away.

Premenstrual syndrome

Premenstrual syndrome or PMS is a disorder that affects menstruating women. Women who suffer from PMS can have many different physical and emotional symptoms. These changes generally appear after ovulation has occurred. Approximately 30% to 80% of women suffer from mild symptoms of PMS prior to their periods, but only about 3% to 5% of women have PMS symptoms severe enough to interfere with their daily lives. Certain risk factors for PMS may include age (late 20s to mid 30s), family history of PMS, and a past history of psychiatric illness. There are many questions as to why PMS occurs. Some people theorize it has to do with hormones produced during the cycle and with **neurotransmitters**, another substance that is produced by the body.

Symptoms of PMS include:

- bloating/weight gain
- food craving
- gastrointestinal problems
- swollen/tender breasts
- sadness/depression
- muscle/joint pain
- headaches/migraines
- overeating
- impulsiveness
- anger/tension
- mood swings
- anxiety
- sleep problems
- fatigue

Treatment

Treatment for PMS includes antidepressant agents, hormonal regimens, and lifestyle changes. Some hormonal regimens, however, may cause symptoms to worsen. Lifestyle changes that may help lessen the symptoms of PMS include exercising, decreasing caffeine intake, increasing **calcium** intake to 1,000 mg/day or 1,200 mg/day, taking from 50 mg/day to 100 mg/day of **vitamin B_6**, and reducing stress.

Your doctor can help you determine if you suffer from PMS. This disorder must be distinguished from other medical and psychiatric disorders that can affect women.

Painful Periods

Painful periods

Pelvic pain can occur at any time throughout a woman's life. It is normal to have some discomfort during the menstrual cycle. Usually, over-the-counter medications known as nonsteroidals are adequate to treat the pain. But pain can be worse during the cycle or can also occur between periods. **Dysmenorrhea** is the medical term used to describe painful menstrual cycles.

There are many reasons for pelvic pain. The female reproductive organs can be involved with pelvic pain, but so can other organs that are located near the pelvis. Problems with the urinary and gastrointestinal tracts can cause discomfort similar to pelvic pain. Sometimes, if a woman has been physically abused or raped, she may suffer from pelvic pain. We'll discuss some of the common problems that can cause pelvic pain.

Uterine fibroids

Fibroids, also known as **leiomyomas**, are benign (noncancerous) muscle tumors of the uterus. Fibroids are composed of smooth muscle cells and are quite common. They are so common that by age 40, approximately 40% of all women may develop fibroids.

There are many locations where fibroids can grow. **Submucosal fibroids** are found under the lining of the uterus. **Intramural fibroids** are located in the muscle wall of the uterus. **Subserosal fibroids** are located under the covering of the uterus (known as the **serosa**). **Pedunculated fibroids** hang off the uterus like mushrooms.

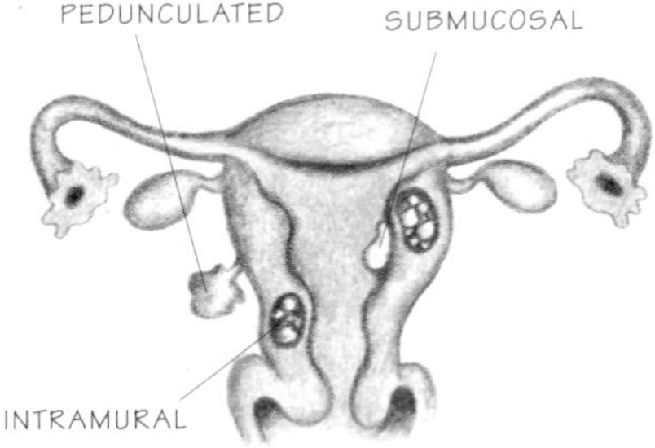

PEDUNCULATED
SUBMUCOSAL
INTRAMURAL

Fibroids depend on estrogen to grow and will continue to grow as long as a woman produces estrogen throughout her menstrual cycle. Symptoms of uterine fibroids can include irregular uterine bleeding as well as pelvic pain. Fibroids can be diagnosed by your doctor during a pelvic exam. The uterus may feel enlarged or irregularly shaped. A pelvic ultrasound can also diagnose fibroids, their size and location. Treatments for fibroids include both hormonal medications and surgery.

Endometriosis

Endometriosis is when cells similar to the lining of the uterus are found outside the uterus. The most common sites for endometriosis are on the **ovaries** and on the **uterosacral ligaments**. These ligaments are located behind the uterus. Implants of endometriosis can be found anywhere in the **pelvis**. They can also occur on the **bowel** and other abdominal organs. Women with endometriosis suffer from pain, mainly during their periods. These implants cycle much like the lining of the uterus does.

A woman who has endometriosis may also experience pain between periods or during intercourse and may have tenderness in her pelvic organs on physical exam.

Endometriosis may be difficult to see on a pelvic ultrasound because the implants are generally quite small. Some women can develop **endometriomas,** which are cysts of endometriosis on the ovaries. These can be seen on a pelvic ultrasound.

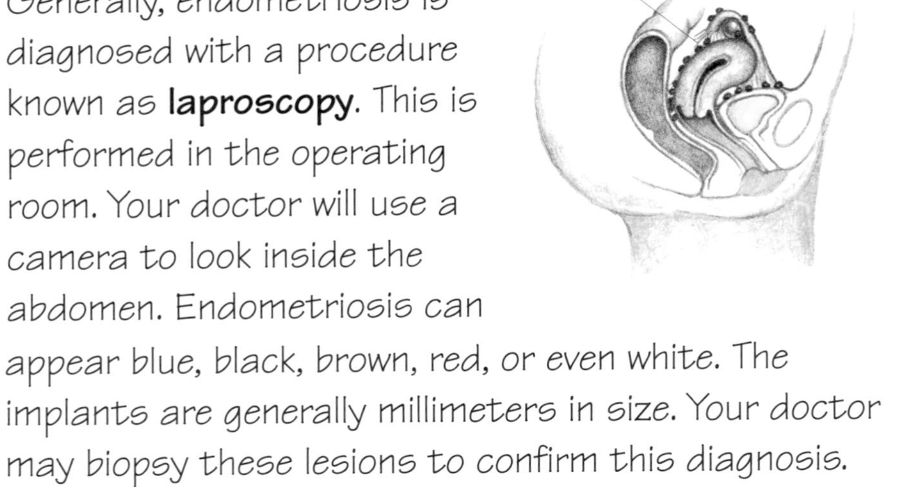

Generally, endometriosis is diagnosed with a procedure known as **laproscopy**. This is performed in the operating room. Your doctor will use a camera to look inside the abdomen. Endometriosis can appear blue, black, brown, red, or even white. The implants are generally millimeters in size. Your doctor may biopsy these lesions to confirm this diagnosis.

Laproscopy can also be used for treatment. Your doctor can **cauterize** (or burn) the implants with laser, heat, or a mild electrical current. Your doctor may even remove the implants surgically. There are also hormonal treatments for endometriosis.

Your doctor can determine which treatment is right for you — either surgical or hormonal.

Pelvic adhesions

Adhesions are present when organs or tissues are "stuck" together. Adhesions can form when a woman has had prior surgery, prior infection, and even endometriosis. Adhesions can cause pain in the pelvic area. This pain occurs because the organs are not able to move like they should.

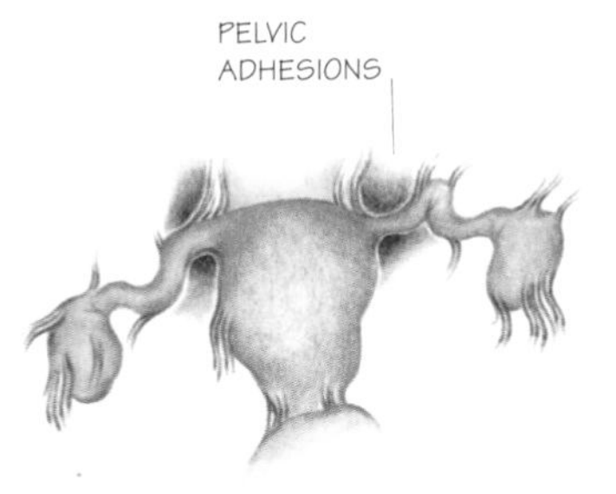

Treatment for adhesions may be surgical. If pain is tolerable with medication, a woman may not need surgery. Adhesions may be diagnosed and/or treated with **laproscopy**.

Cysts

Ovarian cysts

Many different types of cysts on the ovaries can lead to pelvic pain. Most ovarian cysts are benign or noncancerous. In rare cases, they can be cancerous.

Functional cysts

Functional cysts are common, benign cysts that can be found on the ovary at any time during a woman's menstrual cycle. Functional cysts relate to the cycling of the eggs, which compete for ovulation. For a variety of reasons, these cysts may cause pain, usually during ovulation. The pain is generally mild and may go away on its own.

Vaginal Infections

Vaginal infections

There are 3 primary vaginal infections that can cause problems in women. The common symptom of each is a vaginal discharge. Infections can also cause vaginal irritation. Each type of infection is a little different from the others. Let's take a closer look.

Yeast vaginitis

This is also known as a **yeast infection**. Many women will suffer from a yeast infection at some point in their lifetimes. Yeast is caused by a fungus known as **Candida**. Symptoms of a yeast infection include vaginal itching, heavy white discharge, and possible redness of the skin of the vagina and vulva. A yeast infection occurs when the normal flora of a woman's vagina is altered in some way. Every woman

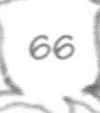

has bacteria that reside in the vagina to keep it healthy. When these bacteria are altered in some way, women can develop yeast infections or even bacterial infections. A yeast infection can be diagnosed by your doctor during a physical examination. Treatment for yeast infections includes antifungal creams or pills. A woman can help prevent yeast infections by using mild soaps, avoiding heavy deodorant products (tampons, pads, etc.), and wearing cotton underwear.

Bacterial vaginosis (BV)

This infection is caused by bacteria known as ***Gardnerella vaginalis***. It occurs for the same reasons a yeast infection occurs. Symptoms of BV include a gray-white discharge along with an odor. Some women may experience irritation of the vagina.

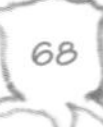

Diagnosis of BV can be made during a physical exam by your doctor. Treatment for BV includes antibiotics, pills, or creams. Sometimes a woman's partner may need to be treated if a woman has recurrent bacterial vaginosis infections. The preventive steps for future BV infections are similar to those for yeast infections.

Trichomonas vaginalis

This vaginal infection is caused by an organism known as a trichomonad. It causes a discharge from the vagina which can be yellow and heavy. Diagnosis can be made during a physical examination. Treatment involves taking antibiotics. A woman and her partner must be treated at the same time to prevent reinfection because trichomonas is also a sexually transmitted disease.

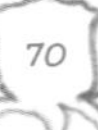

Sexually Transmitted Diseases

Sexually transmitted diseases

Passed through intercourse, these diseases can lead to serious illness in women and in men. A woman can be infected with these diseases and not even know because many of the diseases do not cause outward symptoms.

Gonorrhea

Gonorrhea is caused by bacteria known as **Neisserea gonorrhea**. This disease can cause a yellow discharge. Some women may not have any symptoms. Gonorrhea can be diagnosed with a culture of the cervix. The treatment for gonorrhea is antibiotics.

Some women can develop **pelvic inflammatory disease (PID)** if gonorrhea is left untreated.

Symptoms of PID are tenderness or pain in the uterus and a yellow discharge. Some women may experience a fever. PID can lead to problems with fertility, so a woman should be tested and treated immediately if she thinks she may have gonorrhea.

Chlamydia

This is an infection caused by bacteria known as ***Chlamydia trachomatis***. Again, most women (about 70%) do not have any symptoms with chlamydia. If a woman has symptoms, they include a watery or yellow discharge or pain with urination. Chlamydia can be diagnosed by your doctor taking a culture from the cervix. It is treated with antibiotics. Like gonorrhea, chlamydia can lead to PID if left untreated.

Syphilis

This infection may, if untreated, progress through 3 stages. **Primary syphilis** shows up as a painless, ulcerative lesion on the vulvar area. This lesion appears 1 to 3 weeks after infection occurs. It may go unnoticed in a woman because the ulcer disappears.

About 1 to 3 months after the ulcer goes away, **secondary syphilis** can develop. This can appear like a rash on the palms of the hands and the soles of the feet. Hair loss can also occur, as well as bumps or lesions in the vulvar area.

Tertiary syphilis occurs 15 years or more after infection if syphilis is left untreated. This can cause severe problems with the brain and heart. Syphilis is diagnosed through blood tests and is treated with antibiotics. The earlier the treatment, the fewer doses of antibiotics you would need. If left untreated, syphilis can be life-threatening many years after infection occurs.

Herpes simplex virus (HSV)

With this sexually-transmitted virus, a woman may experience symptoms of burning in the vaginal and vulvar area. She may also experience burning with urination. Blisters can develop in the vulvar area or buttocks. These blisters can be quite painful. Some women may not have symptoms with their first herpes outbreak. **Once infected, a woman will have HSV for life.**

The virus lives in the nerves of the pelvis. Outbreaks of symptoms can occur in no specific pattern.

HSV can be diagnosed with a culture of a visible lesion. If there is not a visible lesion, HSV may be difficult to diagnose. Antiviral medications taken daily can help prevent outbreaks. A person can take antiviral medications for a current outbreak to decrease the duration and intensity of symptoms.

Human immunodeficiency virus (HIV)

This virus can eventually lead to **AIDS (acquired immune deficiency syndrome)**. HIV is sexually transmitted, but it can also be transmitted through blood products, through sharing contaminated needles, through blood-to-blood exposure, and from a pregnant mother to her baby. There is currently no cure. Many medications are available to slow down the evolution of HIV to AIDS.

Women who are infected with HIV may have no symptoms at all. Some people may experience a flu-like illness. If a woman is concerned that she may have had sexual contact with a person who has HIV, she should have a blood test taken. Because a blood test may not be positive until 6 months after infection, the woman should take precautions to prevent potentially infecting others. She should also repeat her blood test in 6 months. It generally takes many, many years for an HIV-positive person to develop AIDS.

Combinations of medications are available to try to prolong this progression or prevent AIDS. You must contact your doctor immediately if you find you are infected with HIV.

Prevention

Sexually transmitted diseases can be prevented. Abstinence is the best way to prevent sexually transmitted diseases. **Abstinence** is the choice not to have sex. If you are not going to practice abstinence, then always practice safe sexual habits. This means proper condom use and making sure that you are aware of your partner's sexual history.

Birth Control

Abstinence

The most important point to understand about birth control is that **abstinence**, not having sexual intercourse, is the best form of birth control. It is 100% effective. If you choose not to practice abstinence and do not want to become pregnant, then birth control is something you must think about as long as you continue to have menstrual cycles.

Barrier methods

These birth control methods include the **diaphragm, cervical cap**, and **female and male condoms**. The effectiveness of these methods is about 80% to 94%. The only barrier methods that offer protection against sexually transmitted diseases and HIV are the male and female condoms. All these methods must be used properly to be effective. If they are used incorrectly, their effectiveness declines. Your doctor should go over specific instructions for proper use with all barrier methods.

Diaphragm

The diaphragm fits in the vagina. It blocks sperm from getting through the cervix and into the uterus. The diaphragm must be fitted by your doctor.

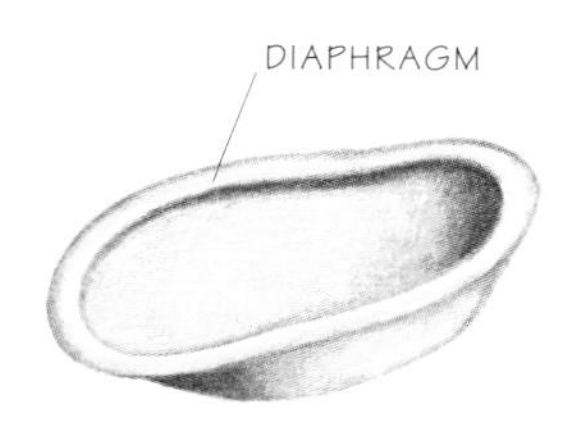

Cervical cap

The cervical cap is similar to a diaphragm but is much smaller and fits specifically over the cervix. Like the diaphragm the cervical cap needs to be fitted by your doctor.

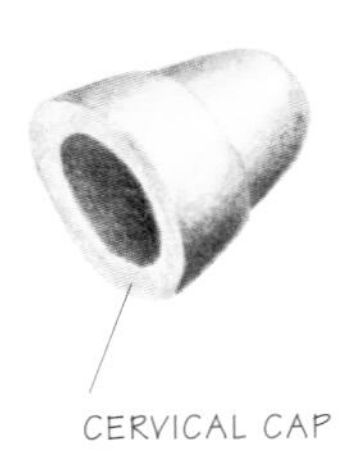

CERVICAL CAP

Condoms

The female condom fits into the vagina and assumes the form of the vagina. This condom prevents sperm from getting into the uterus.

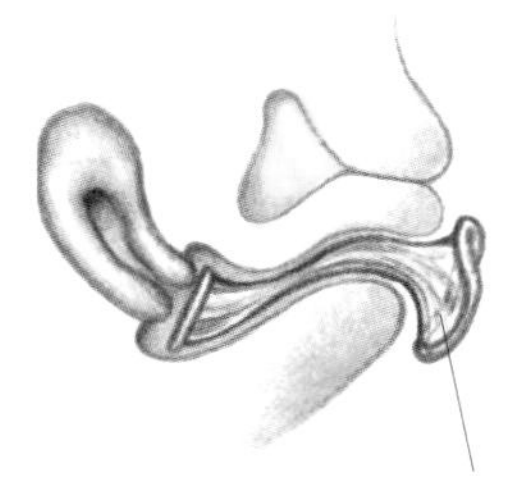

The male condom fits over the penis and prevents sperm from getting into the uterus. Male condoms are available that contain spermicidal lubricants.

Birth control pills (BCPs)

This type of birth control is a method of hormonal contraception. The hormones used in BCPs are estrogen and progesterone. There are also progesterone-only birth control pills. One of the ways birth control works is by preventing ovulation. The pills must be prescribed by your doctor. They must be taken every day. The effectiveness of birth control pills for

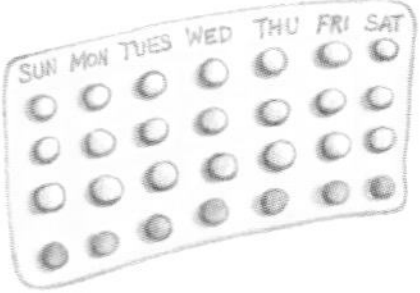

BIRTH CONTROL PILLS

pregnancy prevention is anywhere from 95% to 98% depending on the type of pill used. BCPs do not protect against sexually transmitted diseases. Many women take birth control pills for other female problems including painful periods, heavy periods, and irregular periods, to name a few.

Side effects of birth control pills include irregular uterine bleeding, irritability, bloating, nausea, and breast tenderness. Sometimes the pill can cause migraines or make gallbladder problems worse.

The major complications of BCPs are the increased risks of stroke or blood clots in the lungs or legs. These are rare complications. Certain women may not be able to take birth control pills. Absolute contraindications to the pill include the following:

- Women, age 35 and older, who smoke
- A history of blood clots or active blood clotting disease
- Breast cancer
- Liver disease
- Pregnancy

Other medical conditions require you to get approval from your doctor before you take birth control pills. These include migraine headaches, epilepsy, diabetes, hypertension, and gallbladder problems. Birth control pills may make these problems worse.

You must speak with your doctor to know if birth control pills are right for you.

Long-acting methods

One of these birth control methods includes injectable progesterone. This comes in a shot form and is given every 3 months.

Another form fits under the skin of the arm. It consists of implants of progesterone that work via time release. The implants stay in place for 5 years.

These methods are about 98% to 99% effective. They mainly work by preventing ovulation.

Some of the side effects of the long-acting progesterone methods can include irregular bleeding, headaches, and irritability. You must discuss these methods with your doctor to see which is right for you.

Intrauterine device (IUD)

This is exactly what it sounds like. The IUD is a device that fits into the uterus. Certain IUDs can be changed every year, while others can stay inside the uterus from 6 to 8 years to provide contraception. The IUD is inserted by your doctor. The effectiveness of the IUD is 97% to 99%.

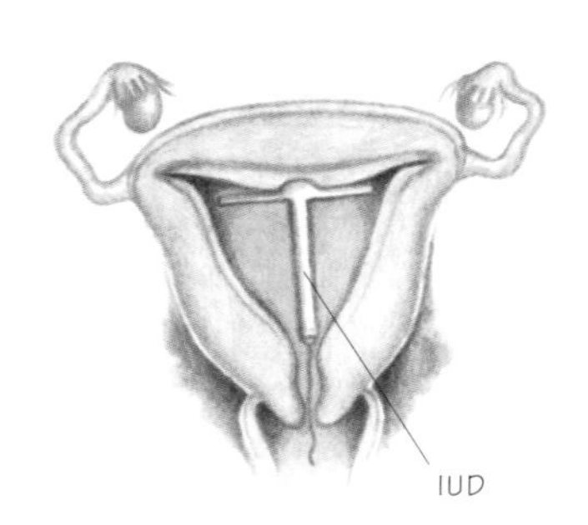

The IUD is **spermicidal**, which means it kills sperm so the sperm cannot reach the egg. Some of the side effects of the IUD include heavier and more painful periods. Risks of the IUD, including infection and perforation of the uterus, are infrequent. Some women may not be candidates for IUDs, so you should discuss this with your doctor.

Surgical methods

The two primary surgical methods of birth control are **tubal ligation** and **vasectomy**. **Tubal ligation** is the permanent female surgical sterilization while **vasectomy** is the permanent male surgical sterilization. Both procedures are 98% to 99% effective.

A tubal ligation is a permanent procedure. The failure rate of tubal ligation varies between 8/1,000 to 30/1,000 women. This means that up to 30 of every 1,000 women

who have this procedure will have an unexpected pregnancy. The risk of tubal pregnancy increases to 50% if the tubal ligation fails. A tubal ligation can be performed surgically after a woman gives birth or during a Caesarean section. A tubal ligation can also be performed through a laprascopic procedure. Besides failure of the procedure, other surgical risks of tubal ligation include bleeding, infection, damage to local organs with need for secondary surgery, and typical anesthesia risks.

Breast Cancer

What is cancer?

Our bodies reproduce cells through cell division. Cells go through **cell differentiation**, which determines which cells will perform each specialized function within the body. Life is like a puzzle. The cells in our bodies grow and fit together in a very particular way ...

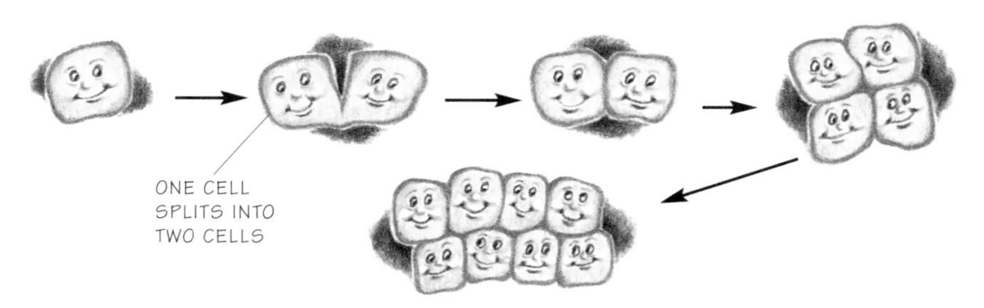

Cancerous cells lack control and pattern. They undergo cell division rapidly without stopping. The result is a crowding of the normal cells. This crowding robs the healthy cells of available nutrients and eventually leads to the death of healthy cells. The puzzle or network of normal cells becomes damaged or interrupted.

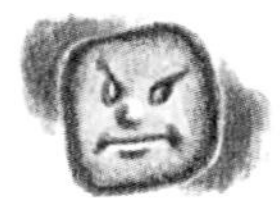

CANCER CELL

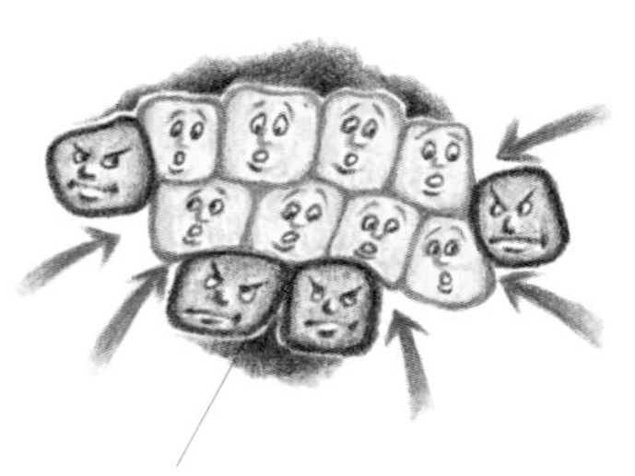

CANCER CELLS CROWDING NORMAL CELLS

The mass of cancerous cells becomes a tumor. These masses can continue to grow and destroy neighboring healthy tissue.

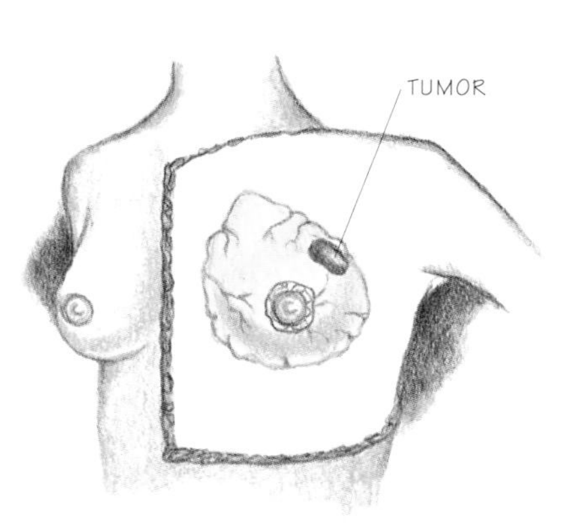

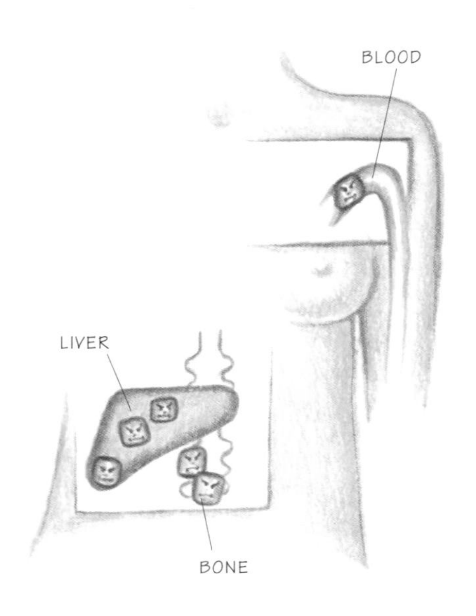

Tumors can also spread, or **metastasize**, to other parts of the body through the blood or lymph system.

Why is screening for cancer so important?

Early detection is the best protection. Cancer may occur in almost any organ of the body, and each type of cancer has its own growth rate. Diagnosis is important to determine the type, location, and extent to which the cancer has spread. The earlier the cancer is diagnosed, the better the woman's chances for survival.

What causes cancer?

Cancer may be caused by multiple factors. **External** factors include chemicals, radiation, viruses, and environment. **Internal** factors include hormones, heredity (family history of cancer in a mother or sister), immune system, and metabolic conditions. No single factor explains why cancer growth occurs.

What are the risk factors for breast cancer?

Just because you have one or more of the following risk factors does not mean you will eventually develop breast cancer. It means you must be especially aware of your body and have routine screenings for breast cancer.

Certain risk factors may increase your chances of developing breast cancer:

- Significant family history, especially mother or sister
- Failure to ovulate or release an egg regularly (irregular periods)
- Age at menopause older than 55
- Obesity, diabetes, high-fat diet
- Never having children
- Having your first child after age 30
- Unusual cells found in a breast lump
- Excessive alcohol consumption
- Early menarche

Signs and symptoms of breast cancer

These include a lump in the breast, discharge from the nipple — especially green or red, change in the shape of one or both breasts, indentation of breast skin or "peau de orange" that resembles dimpling, or redness of breast skin.

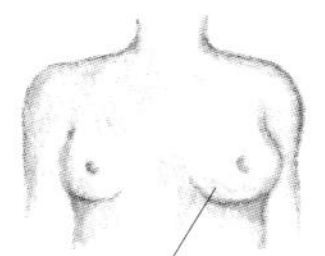

ENLARGED BREAST

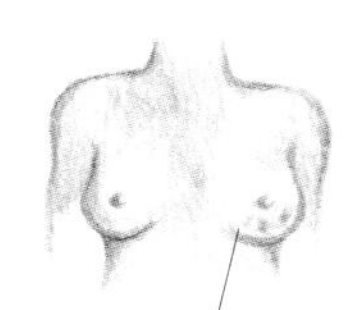

DIMPLING OF THE BREAST

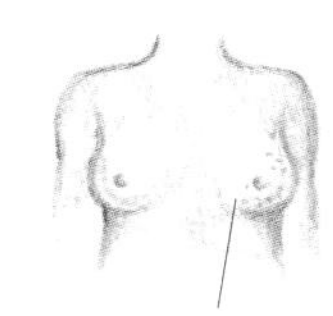

REDNESS OF BREAST SKIN

Routine screening for breast cancer is very important. It begins with self-examination starting at age 20. **Every woman should check her breasts monthly**. The best time for this is a week after your period begins. If you no longer menstruate, you should pick the same time every month.

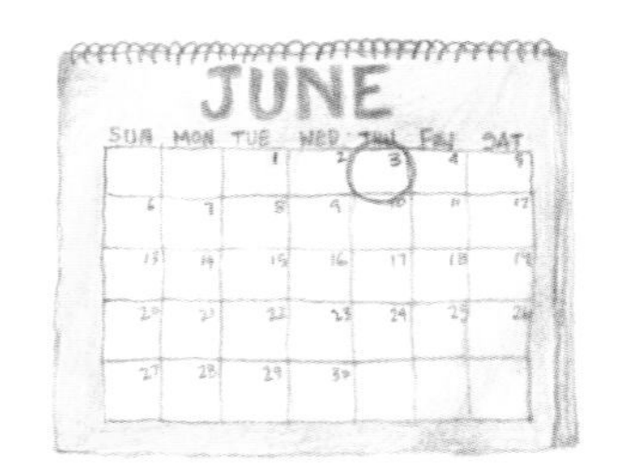

Your doctor should examine your breasts every year.

A breast self-exam is performed using your fingertips. You should start feeling **under your arm** and go around your breast in a circular motion. You should feel from under your collarbone to your breastbone. This should be done on both sides.

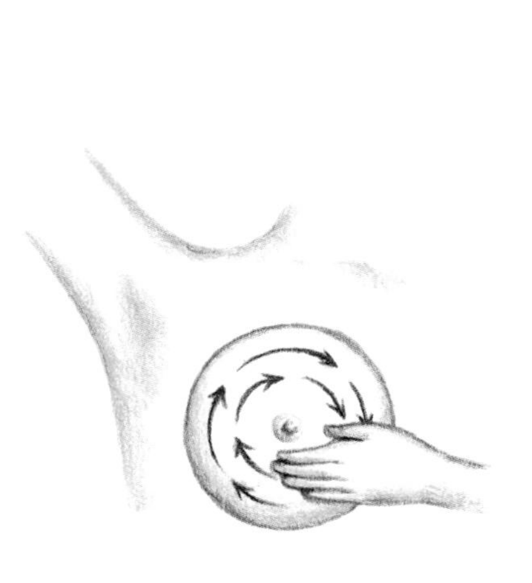

A convenient time to do a self-examination may be when you are taking a shower.

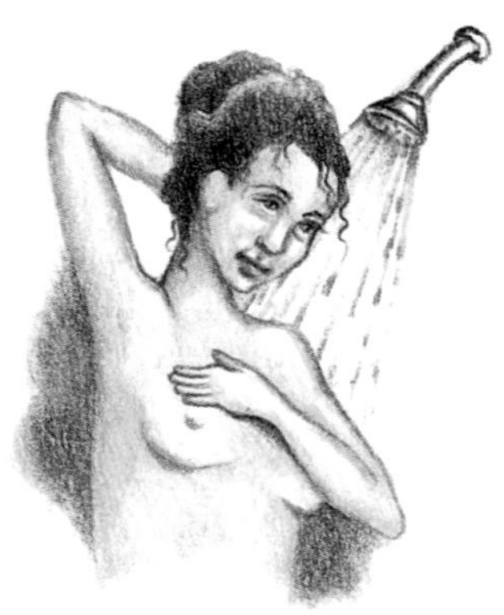

Always look at your breasts in the mirror. You should also squeeze your breasts from the bottom to check for discharge from your nipples. If discharge arises from your nipple, you should contact your doctor.

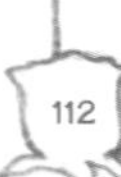

What if I feel a lump or my doctor feels a lump? Should I assume I have cancer?

No! Just because you feel a lump, do not assume that it is breast cancer. Lumps can be caused by factors other than cancer. An **abscess**, **inflammation**, **clogged duct**, **cyst**, and **fibroadenoma** are some of the **benign** (noncancerous) conditions that may cause lumps in the breast.

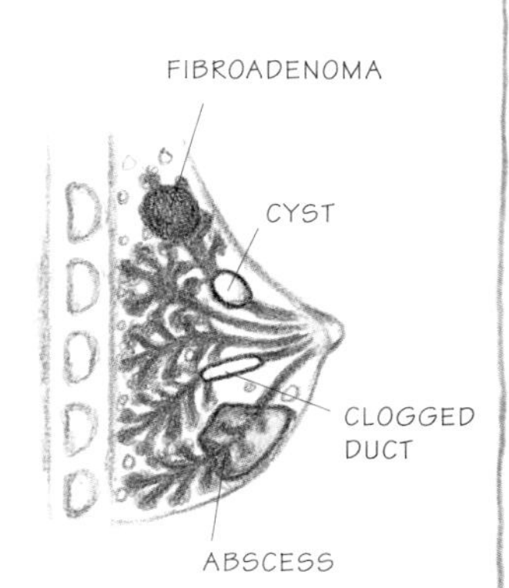

All lumps should be reported to your doctor immediately and checked promptly. You may be asked to get a mammogram. Additionally, an **ultrasound** may be ordered to determine if the lump is fluid-filled or **cystic**.

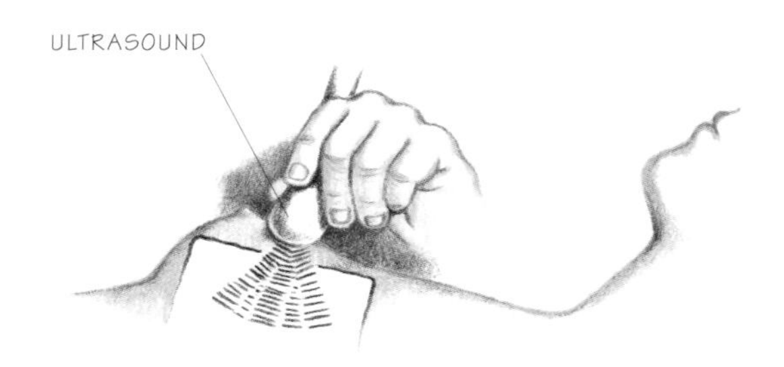

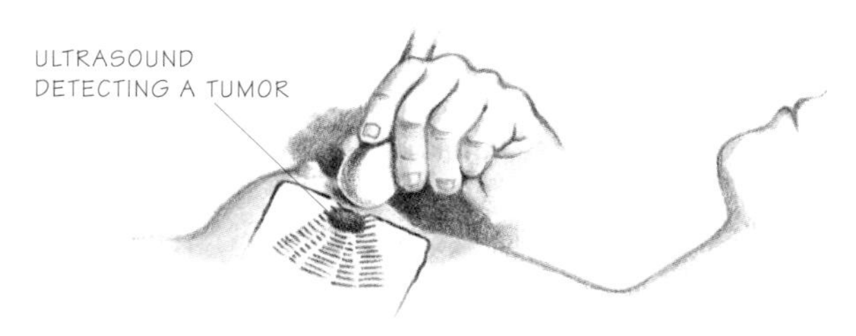

If the lump is only a cyst, the fluid may be removed with a needle and analyzed to determine if it is **malignant** (cancerous). If the lump reappears, if the fluid tested contained malignant cells, or if the lump is not filled with fluid, it may be removed by a method known as a **biopsy**. The biopsy, or lump sample, will also be analyzed for malignancy.

Mammogram

You may not be able to feel a lump smaller than an almond or a pea. This is why a mammogram is so important. It can detect lumps one-tenth of the size that you can feel. A positive mammogram may be a sign, though not proof, that cancer is present.

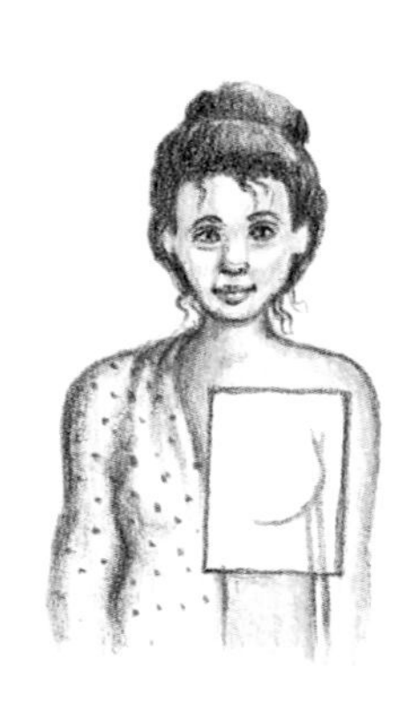

A mammogram is simply an X-ray of your breast. Ordinarily, your first or **baseline** mammogram should be taken between ages 35 and 40 if you have any risk factors. However, it may be done sooner depending on your family history. Unfortunately, mammograms may not be as effective at detecting breast cancer in younger women due to the denseness of the breast tissue. The current recommendation is to get a mammogram every 1 to 2 years, starting at age 40, and every year after age 50. You should talk to your doctor to see when a mammogram is right for you.

Invasive disease

When cancerous cells spread to nearby or underlying tissue, they are considered **invasive.** Invasive breast cancer is often detected as a lump during a breast exam or as a mass on a mammogram.

Breast cancer staging

Cancers are categorized by a process called **staging**. Doctors determine the **stage** of a cancer according to the tumor size, location, and whether it has spread to other organs or lymph nodes. This can be performed through **examination**, **X-rays**, and/or **surgery**, depending on the type of cancer. The different stages affect the prognosis and treatment of a woman who suffers from cancer.

Breast cancer is generally classified into 4 stages. Stage IV is the most advanced cancer as the cancer has spread to other organs.

Treatment

Two types of treatment are typically chosen for breast cancer:

1) **local treatment** — treatment targeted at a specific site

2) **systemic treatment** — treatment throughout the entire body

Several factors influence the type of treatment chosen. The stage of the disease; the size, type, and location of the tumor; your age and physical health; size of breasts; menopausal status; and results of other laboratory tests are all taken into consideration.

Local treatment

Local treatment includes

1) surgery
2) radiation therapy

Stage I and Stage II cancers may be treated with local treatments. In some cases, these treatments will be combined with systemic treatments.

1. Surgery

Women with breast cancer may undergo one of the following types of surgery:

- **lumpectomy** — removing only the breast lump and some surrounding tissue
- **partial** or **segmental mastectomy** — removing the tumor, surrounding tissue, and chest muscle lining
- **total mastectomy** — removing the breast tissue

- **modified radical mastectomy** — removing the breast tissue, some lymph nodes, and chest muscle lining
- **radical mastectomy** — removing the breast tissue, lymph nodes, chest muscle, and surrounding tissue. This procedure is rare.
- **axillary lymph node dissection** — removing lymph nodes in the axillary region for treatment and/or staging purposes.

Possible side effects of surgery include swelling, loss of strength, stiffness, numbness or tingling, bleeding, infection, and/or blood clots.

2. Radiation therapy

High-energy radiation is concentrated on a particular site in an attempt to destroy or control cancerous cell growth. Radiation can come from a machine (external) or from implanted radioactive material (internal). Radiation treatment for the breast is generally external. Other organs affected with cancer may be treated with internal radiation.

External treatment for the breast may occur on a daily basis for a short period of time. This is typically an outpatient procedure. It is usually done in conjunction with a lumpectomy (see page 123).

Systemic treatment

Systemic treatment, which involves chemotherapy, is typically combined with local treatment for Stage III and Stage IV cancers.

With **chemotherapy**, your doctor will use a combination of drugs that enter the bloodstream via the mouth, vein, or muscle. There are many types of chemotherapy. Treatment is performed on an outpatient basis.

Several treatments may be necessary and can be given in cycles:

treatment → recovery,
treatment → recovery, etc.

Possible side effects of chemotherapy include hair loss, nausea, diarrhea, weight loss, dry mouth, and/or infertility.

Oral chemotherapy

SERMS — Selective Estrogen Receptor Modulators — are a class of estrogen-like hormonal medications that have different actions on select tissues. Each medication in this class is somewhat different.

SERMS can affect certain tissues including the breast, bone, and endometrium (lining of the uterus). SERMS are most often used for treatment of breast cancer and osteoporosis.

SERMS can be used to help in the long-term treatment of certain types of breast cancer. Research is also under way to determine what role (if any) SERMS can play in breast cancer prevention.

Side effects of these medications may be similar to menopause, including hot flashes, irregular vaginal bleeding, and vaginal dryness.

Summary

One in 8 women will develop breast cancer. You need to know your risks. You should see your doctor yearly for a breast exam. You also should perform a monthly self-examination. It is very important to work with your doctor to determine what screening is best for you. If you have breast cancer, it is vital to know your treatment options. There are many new treatments on the horizon, so you should consult with your doctor.

Staying Healthy

No smoking

Smoking is bad for your health. Smoking can lead to stress on the cardiovascular system, lung cancer, and emphysema. Smoking has also been linked to abnormal Pap smears and earlier menopause. If a woman is pregnant and smokes, she might experience preterm labor and **intrauterine growth restriction** or low-birthweight babies. Other undesirable effects of smoking are wrinkling of the skin and staining the teeth yellow.

Smoking is bad for the entire cardiovascular system because it:

A) Introduces carbon monoxide into the body

B) Lowers the "good" HDL-cholesterol

A. Carbon monoxide

Oxygen attaches to the red blood cells in the lungs. Red blood cells transport the oxygen throughout the body.

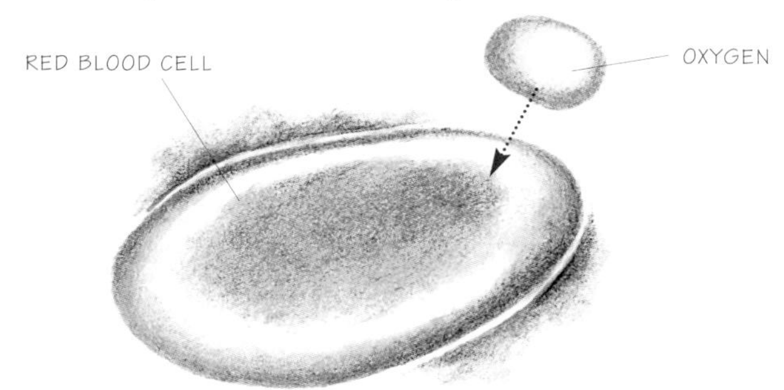

When you smoke, you inhale carbon monoxide into your lungs. Carbon monoxide frequently binds to the red blood cells at the site where oxygen normally binds. Therefore, less oxygen is carried by the blood, and this results in less oxygen available for use throughout the body.

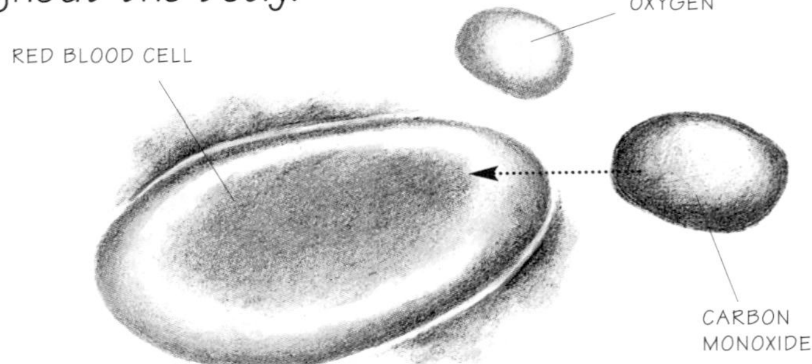

B. Lower HDL-cholesterol

Two other reasons for not smoking are that it reduces the amount of HDL-cholesterol or "good cholesterol" in your bloodstream, and it makes your blood clot more easily, increasing the potential for an arterial blockage (heart attack or stroke).

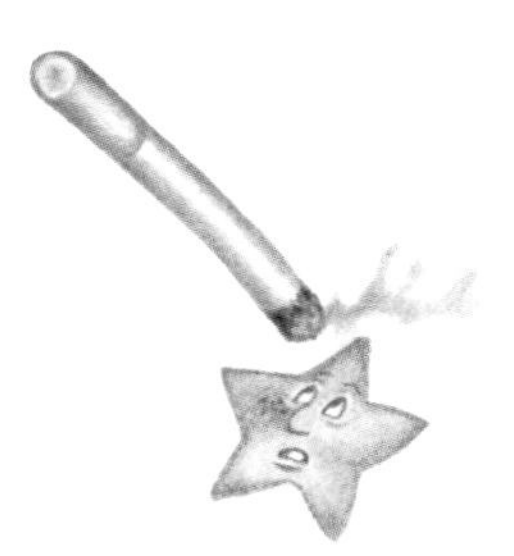

SMOKING REDUCES HDL-CHOLESTEROL

Limited alcohol consumption

Experts agree that excess alcohol consumption over time can lead to many harmful effects, including high blood pressure, cirrhosis of the liver, and damage to the heart. The issue is the balance between **moderate** and **excessive** alcohol consumption. Men should consume no more than 2 drinks* daily, and women, because of their smaller body size, should not consume more than 1 drink* each day. The 7 to 14 allowable

drinks in a week should not be consumed in a few days or during a weekend of binge drinking. People who should not drink include individuals with high levels of triglycerides in their blood (over 300 mg/dL), women who are pregnant, individuals who are under age, people with a genetic predisposition for alcoholism or who are recovering from alcoholism, and those taking certain medications.

***A guide:** One drink is defined as 5 ounces of wine, 12 ounces of beer, or 1-1/2 ounces of 80-proof liquor.

Proper diet

Each person's body handles foods differently. Contact your doctor or hospital for the name of a registered dietitian who can help you plan your diet for your lifestyle and your nutritional needs.

Vitamin D and calcium

All women must get both **vitamin D** and **calcium** in their diets, either through food sources or through supplementation. The proper amounts of vitamin D and calcium can be obtained by eating dairy products, leafy greens, yogurt, nuts, and whole grains.

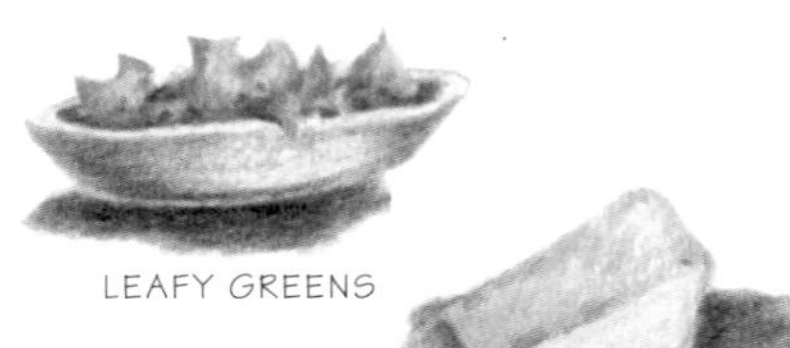

LEAFY GREENS

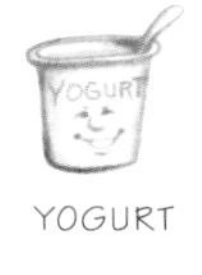

YOGURT

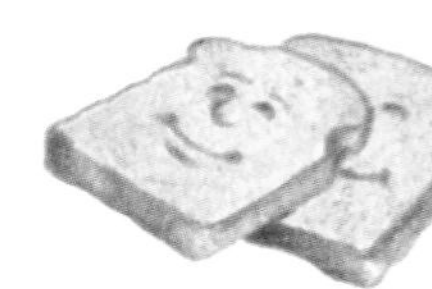

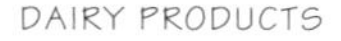

DAIRY PRODUCTS

WHOLE GRAINS

Vitamin D is needed to absorb calcium into the body. Vitamin D is made when the body absorbs sunlight in skin and combines it with a form of cholesterol. Excessive sun exposure may be harmful, but 30 minutes a day is effective in producing sufficient amounts of vitamin D provided that skin is exposed to natural, outdoor sunlight.

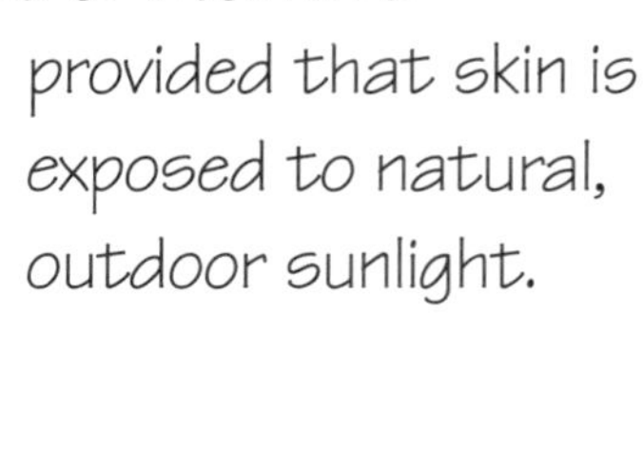

People who live in northern climates of the United States may not achieve adequate sunlight exposure. Contact your doctor to find out if you should take calcium supplements and vitamin D.

Vitamin D can be found in milk and foods like broccoli or salmon. The recommended daily allowance for vitamin D is 400 I.U. An 8-ounce glass of milk contains about 100 I.U. of vitamin D. The vitamin can also be taken as a food supplement.

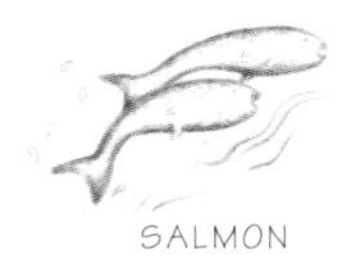
SALMON

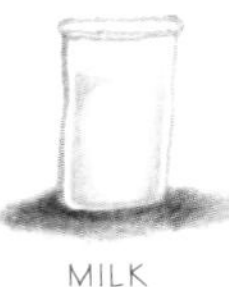

MILK

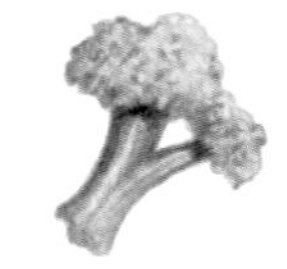
BROCCOLI

Calcium intake

Calcium absorption is at its peak during the bone-building phase of adolescence. After age 65, a woman's body absorbs less than 50% of the needed calcium from food and supplements.

Calcium is an important part of a woman's diet. A calcium supplement is usually needed if a woman does not have **3 to 4 cups** of milk or yogurt each day.

Here are the recommended daily calcium intakes for a woman during various ages of her life:

• Age 11 through age 24	1,200 to 1,500 mg/day
• Pregnancy	1,200 mg/day
• Premenopausal	1,000 mg/day
• Postmenopausal	with HRT* 1,000 mg/day
	without HRT* 1,500 mg/day

*hormone replacement therapy

Calcium carbonate and **calcium citrate** are two very good forms of calcium supplements. However, not all of the calcium or calcium carbonate may be absorbed by the body. Consult your doctor about which supplement is best for you.

Meats

Limit the amount of fatty meats, particularly those foods that are high in saturated fats (bacon, sausage, and prime rib), to 1 or 2 servings per week. Cook meats using little or no fat, such as baking, broiling, grilling, stewing, or stir-frying without adding fat.

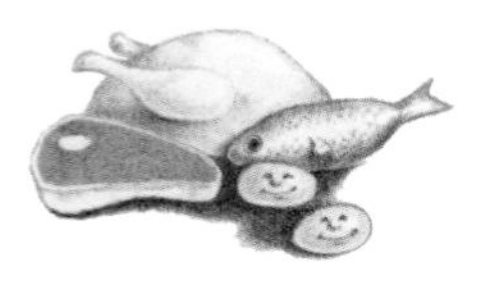

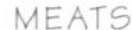

MEATS

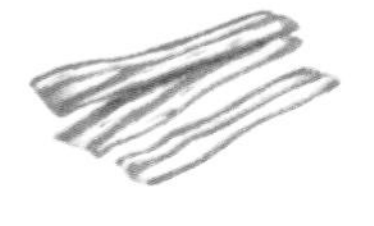

BACON

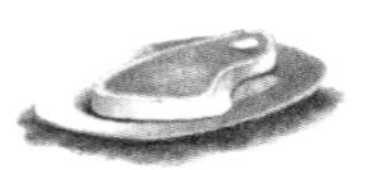

PRIME RIB

Eggs

It used to be thought that these were the main culprits of elevated cholesterol. This may not be true. However, if you have elevated cholesterol or a history of heart disease, you should limit egg yolks to no more than 3 or 4 per week. Egg whites or "egg substitutes" have no cholesterol and do not need to be limited.

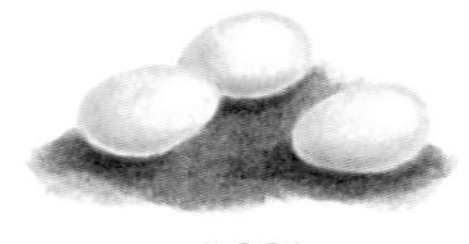

Dairy products

Switch from whole milk to 2% and then to 1% or even skim milk. Use low-fat cheeses, yogurt, and sour cream. For a healthier dessert, look for low-fat ice cream or sherbet.

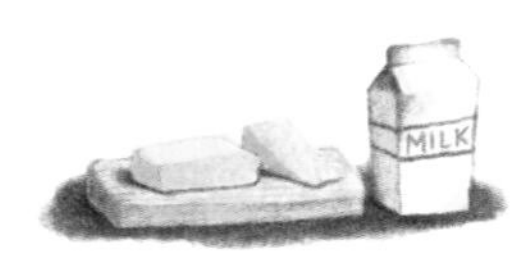

DAIRY PRODUCTS

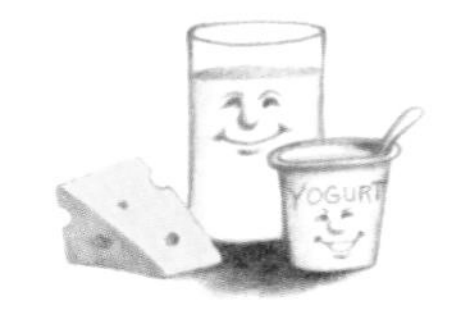

LOW-FAT DAIRY PRODUCTS

Whole grains, fruits, and vegetables

Another thing you can do to help improve your overall diet is to eat healthier foods. The American Heart Association recommends that you try to increase the number of servings of foods that are high in whole grains, such as breads and cereals, and try to have at least **5 servings** of fruits and vegetables every day.

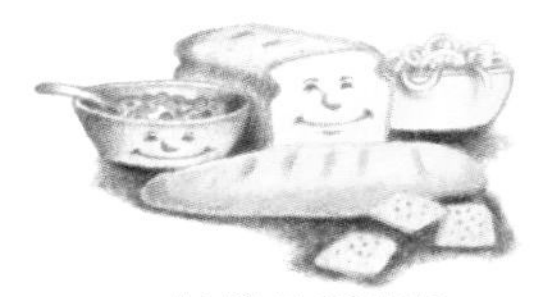

WHOLE GRAINS

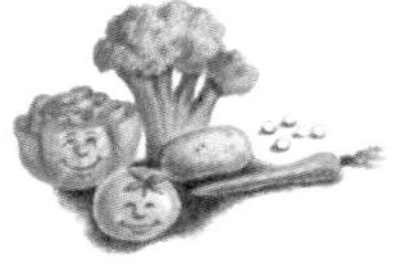

VEGETABLES

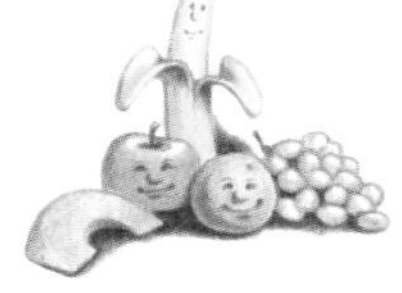

FRUITS

Exercise

Currently, only 22% of adults in the United States exercise at a level that benefits their cardiovascular systems. What are some important considerations?

1) Type of exercise

2) Amount and regularity of exercise

3) Intensity of exercise

1. Type of exercise

Aerobic exercise

To meet your general fitness goals, the best type of exercise is **aerobic** exercise.

Aerobic exercise does not necessarily require special equipment or a health club membership. Aerobic exercises are those that require a lot of oxygen. These exercises include walking, jogging, cycling, swimming, cross-country skiing, or rowing.

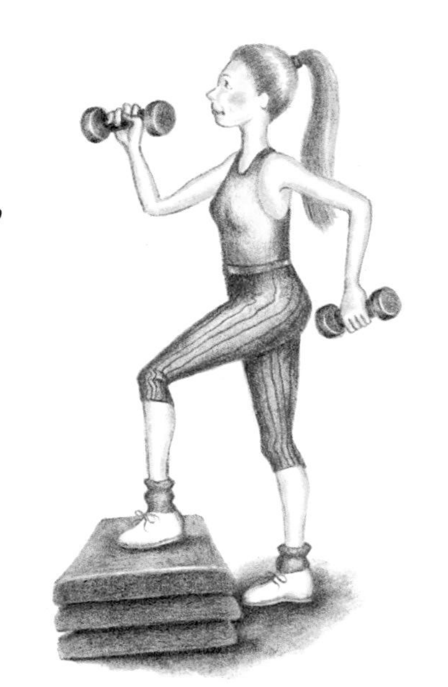

20-30 minutes a day, 5 days a week

2. Amount and regularity of exercise

The U.S. surgeon general recommends that healthy adults exercise 20 to 30 minutes, 5 days a week.

There are nearly 50 half hours in a 24-hour day. Exercising for 30 minutes daily requires **only about 2%** of your total day. Try to find 1, or 2, or 3 exercises you like to do. You'll enjoy the variety.

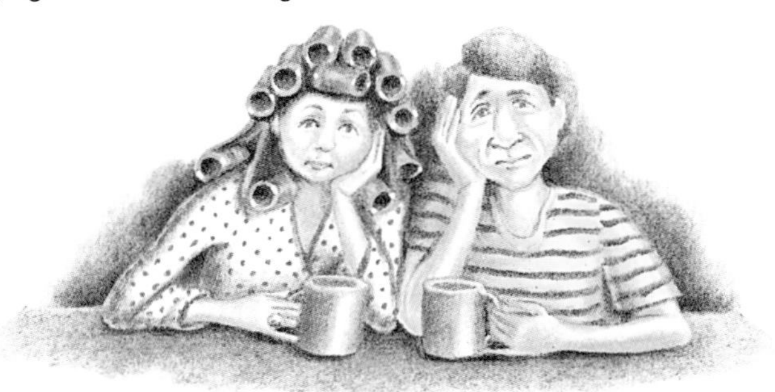

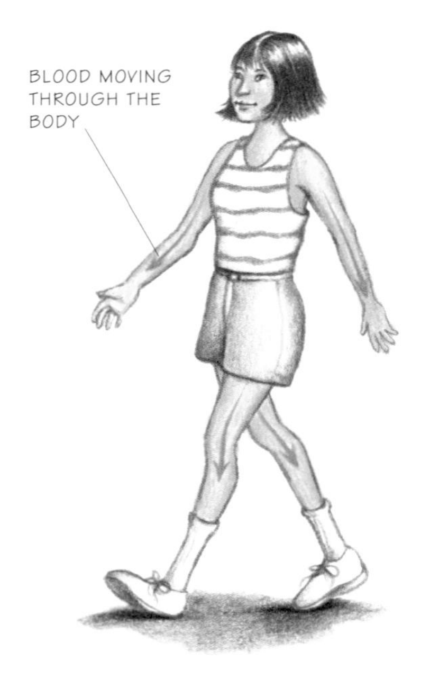

3. Intensity of exercise

Warm up

By walking or cycling slowly, you move the blood out to the working muscles. A warm-up should start slowly and last 5 to 10 minutes.

You cannot maintain "all out" *exercise* (100%) for very long. An *example of* an "all out" *exercise* is sprinting. Actually, you may *only* maintain a sprint for about 15 *seconds.*

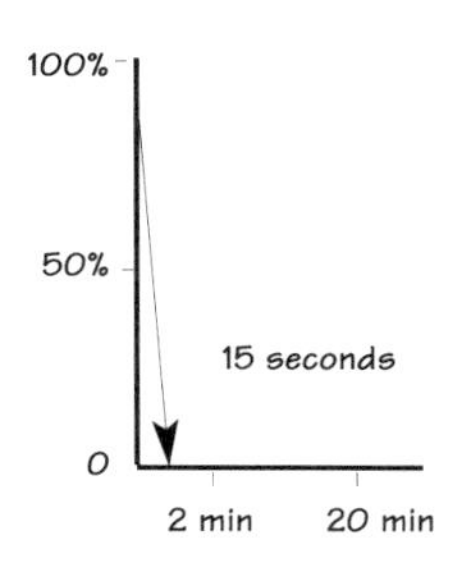

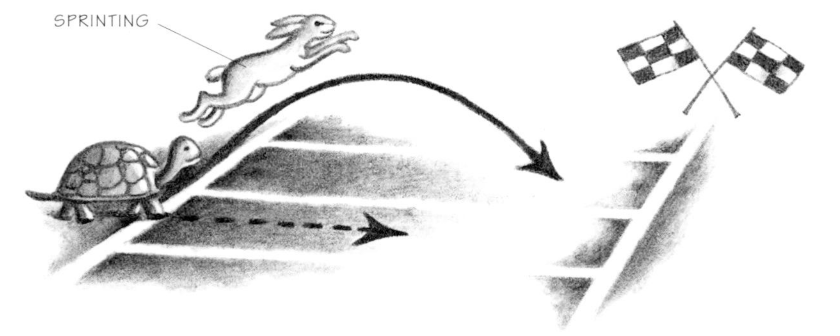

If you slow the exercise down a bit, to about 90%, you may still only go for about 2 minutes!

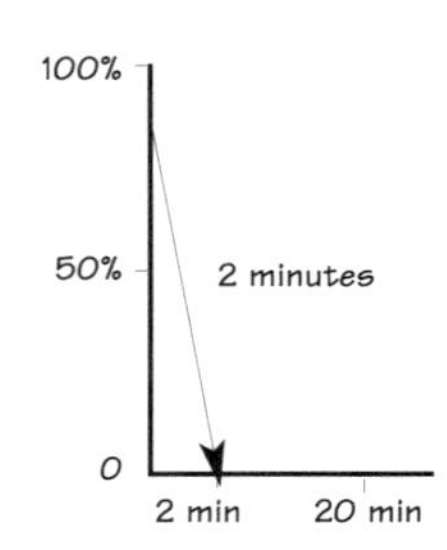

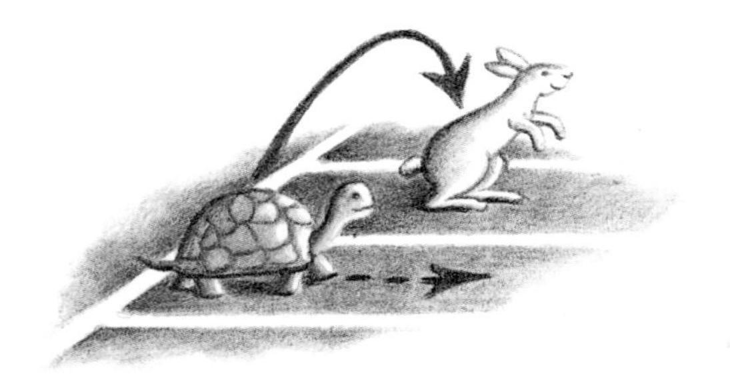

What if you slow your exercise down to 75% or even 50%? There is a **huge** difference. Now you may easily go more than 20 minutes.

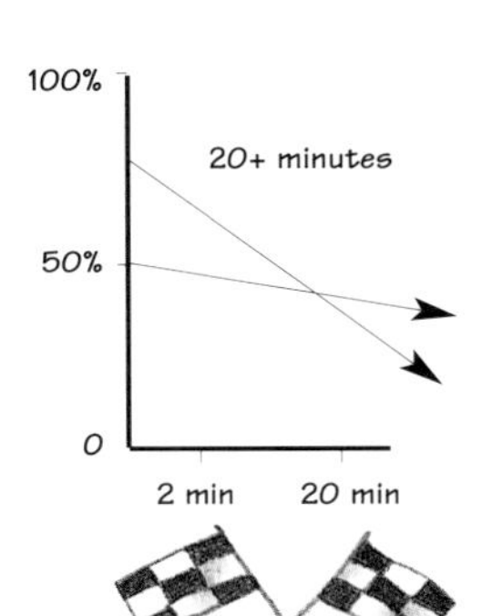

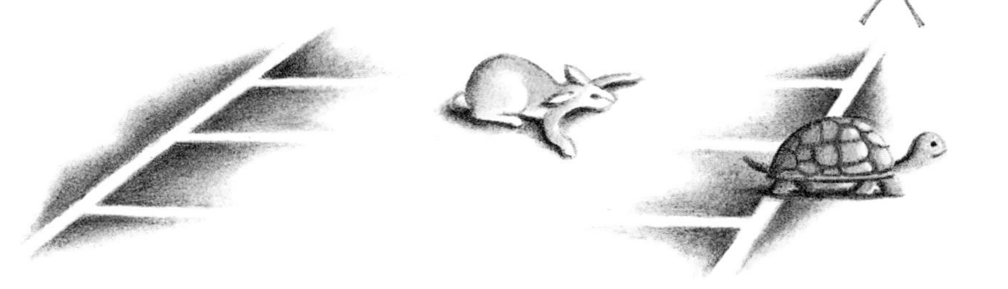

Simply —

By slowing down the pace, you may be able to exercise for a longer period of time.

Many exercise physiologists use the following generally accepted formula to determine the exercise target heart rate of a healthy individual. If you have a history of cardiovascular disease, or if you are just starting a program, **check with your doctor before starting an exercise routine**. Your doctor is aware of the many factors that may need to be considered in modifying your exercise intensity.

Target heart rate example

Your age: 50	**Your resting pulse: 70**
1. 220 minus your age:	1. 220 - 50 = 170
2. Answer #1 minus your resting pulse:	2. 170 - 70 = 100
3. Answer #2 times 0.5:	3. 100 x 0.5 = 50
4. Answer #3 plus your resting pulse:	4. 50 + 70 = 120
5. Answer #2 times 0.75:	5. 100 x 0.75 = 75
6. Answer #5 plus your resting pulse:	6. 75 + 70 = 145
7. **Target heart rate** equals range between values for #4 and #6:	7. **120 to 145 beats per minute, or 12 to 14 beats for 6 seconds**

Now it's your turn

Here is how you determine the heart rate of an apparently healthy individual. Please consult with your doctor to make sure that this is an accurate target heart rate for your condition.

1. Measure your pulse (heart rate) for 60 seconds: ______
2. Take 220 and subtract your age: 220 - ______ = ______
3. Now take the answer in #2 and subtract your pulse: ______
4. Take the answer in #3 and multiply by 0.5: ______
5. Take the answer in #4 and add your pulse: ______
6. Take the answer in #3 and multiply by 0.75: ______
7. Take the answer in #6 and add your pulse: ______
8. Your target heart rate should range from the answer in #5 (______) to the answer in #7 (______).
9. Divide each answer in #8 by 10 to determine your pulse for 6 seconds: ______ to ______ .

How hard and how often should I exercise?

When you are just starting out, try to exercise very comfortably. Here are 4 quick tips.

1) Try to exercise so that you are breathing noticeably but are **not** out of breath. Remember this simple rule: you should be able to carry on a conversation while you are exercising.

2) Sweating is a good thing. This means that your body is working hard enough and receiving the necessary stimulus for the muscles and the heart.

3) If you are not fatigued and are completely recovered from exercising on the previous day, then you should exercise **daily**.

4) Give yourself a **warm-up** before exercise (several minutes of easy walking) and a **cooldown** at the end of exercise (again, several minutes of easy walking). Ask an exercise specialist for some recommendations for stretching after your workout, and discuss the intensity of the exercise with your doctor.

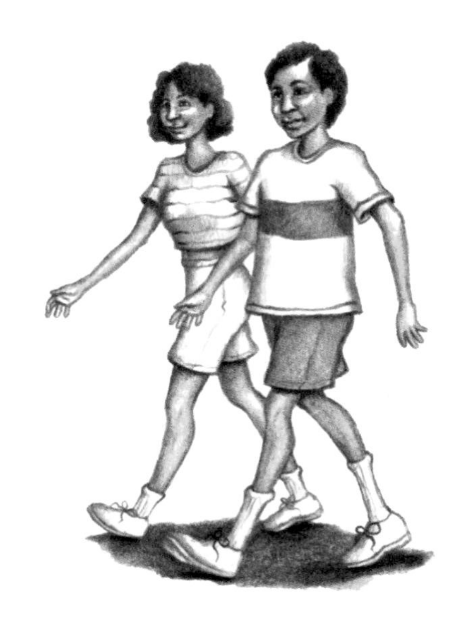

If you are just starting an exercise program, probably the simplest exercise to try is walking. It is fairly easy to do for 20 minutes. Check with your doctor for additional input on your exercise program.

VERY, VERY important

Cool down. As important as the warm-up and the aerobic exercise are to improving your fitness, you must also include a cooldown as part of your exercise routine.

Your cooldown should be just like your warm-up. At the end of your exercise routine, give yourself 5 to 10 minutes of nice, easy walking. You also may want to include some mild stretching.

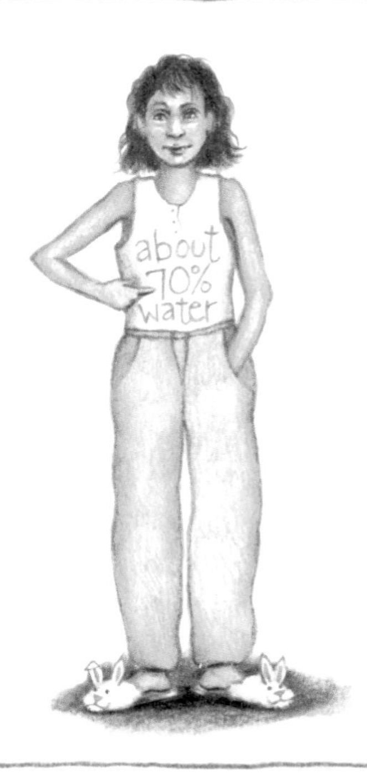

Another consideration — water

Water is needed for virtually *every* function of the body. The body is approximately 70% water.

During the course of the day, you lose water through sweating, breathing, and waste. Replacement of water (rehydration) is important — especially when participating in an exercise program. A prudent recommendation is that you should drink 6 to 10 glasses of water per day. Sorry, caffeinated drinks and alcohol do not count. They are "diuretics," meaning that they actually may cause you to lose even more water.

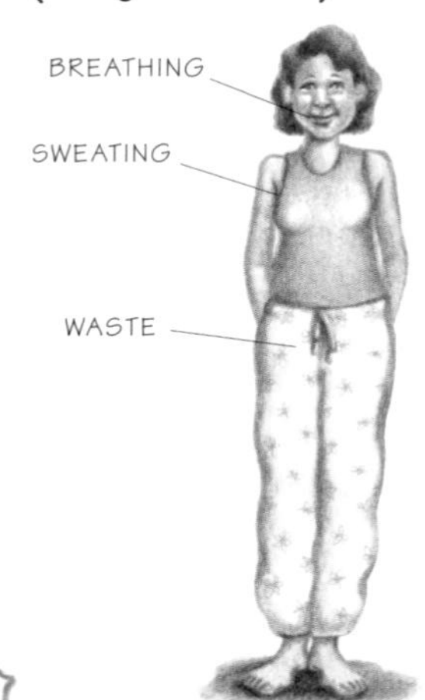

Maintaining physical and spiritual health

Maintaining physical and spiritual health can help improve your quality of life. Exercise is one of the most important behaviors you can adopt to help maintain your physical health. Eating the proper diet is also vital. Getting annual physical examinations from your doctor can help screen for illness and can also help cure or treat any medical illnesses you may have.

Spiritual and mental health are also important to help decrease stress in your life. When you are under stress, your brain releases signals to the body through the nerves. These signals allow your body to respond to various situations. Undue stress can lead to anxiety, depression, and tension. It can also lead to irregularities in your menstrual cycle and can affect your cardiovascular system.

A woman can reduce stress by practicing meditation, doing deep breathing exercises, praying, listening to music, or even going for a walk. Whatever you find relaxing is what you should do **every day** to relieve stress in your life.

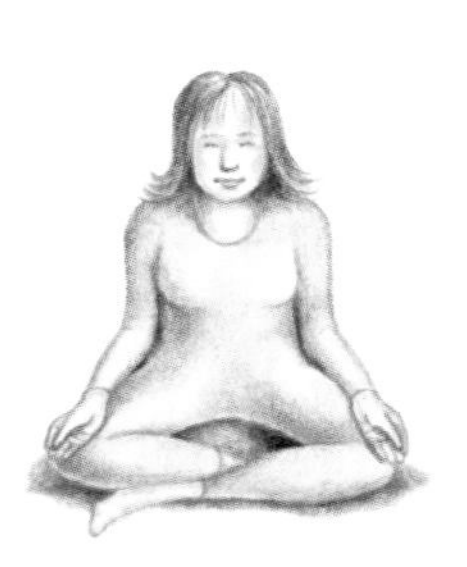

MEDITATION

Questions

Here are some questions that you may want to take with you the next time you go to see your doctor.

Based on my weight, blood pressure, and blood cholesterol level, should I talk to someone about changing my diet?

Yes **No**

Contact your local hospital for the name of a registered dietitian.

Dietitian ______________________________

Address ______________________________

____

Phone ______________________________

How often should I have a Pap smear?

Answer

Do I need to get a mammogram? How often?

Answer

What treatment is best for me if I have breast cancer?

Answer ____

____

____

____

____

Woman to Woman ...

We hope that you have found this book informative and useful. We hope that if you feel something is going on with your body you will tell your doctor about it right away. It is **so important** to keep your body and your mind healthy. We want to help you understand your body and what you can do to maintain the best health possible. Remember how important you are to yourself and to those loved ones who surround you. Please remember to take the time to take care of yourself. You are a very special woman!

Bibliography

American Cancer Society on breast cancer at http://www3.cancer.org accessed February 1999.

American Cancer Society Recommendations Screening Mammogram. Facts and Figures. July 1998.

American College of Obstetrics and Gynecology Technical Bulletin. "Chronic Pelvic Pain." May 1996: Number 223.

American College of Obstetrics and Gynecology Technical Bulletin. "Hormone Replacement Therapy." April 1992: 166.

American College of Obstetrics and Gynecology Technical Bulletin. "Sterilization." April 1996: Number 222.

American College of Sports Medicine position stand. "The Recommended Quality and Quantity of Exercise for Developing and Maintaining Cardiorespiratory and Muscular Fitness in Healthy Adults." *Medicine and Science in Sports and Exercise* April 1990.

The American Journal of Managed Care Special Report. Creating an Optimal Strategy of Treating Endometriosis and Chronic Pelvic Pain. May 1999. Volume 5. Number 5. Suppl.

Association of Professors of Obstetrics and Gynecology Educational Series on Women's Health Issues. "Contraception." Feb. 1999.

Association of Professors of Obstetrics and Gynecology Educational Series on Women's Health Issues. "Osteoporosis, Treatment, Monitoring." 1996.

Association of Professors of Obstetrics and Gynecology Educational Series on Women's Health Issues. "Premenstrual Syndrome and premenstrual dysphoric disorder: Syncope, diagnosis and treatment." Oct. 1998.

Baker, V.D., and R.B. Jaffe. "Clinical uses of antiestrogens." *Obstetric Gynecological Survey* Jan. 1995: 45-49.

Cogswell, M.E. "Nicotine Withdrawal Symptoms." *North Carolina Medical Journal* 1 Jan. 1995: 40-45.

The Contraception Report. 5 Patient Update. Nov. 1998. Volume 9. No. 5.

Cummings, S., and M.C. Nevitt, W.S. Browner, K. Stone, K.M. Fox, K.E. Ensrud, J. Cauley, D. Black, T.M. Vogt for The Study of Osteoporotic Fractures Research Group. "Risk factors for hip fractures in white women." *New England Journal of Medicine* 23 March 1995.

Delmas, P.D., et al. "Effects of raloxifene on bone mineral density, serum cholesterol concentrations, and uterine endometrium in postmenopausal women." *New England Journal of Medicine* 4 Dec. 1997: 1641-1647.

Dialogues in Contraception. Contraceptive Selection in Women with Medical Conditions. Summer 1999. Volume 5. Number 7.

Eckel, R.H. "Obesity in Heart Disease." *Circulation* 1997: 3248-3250.

Fernando, G.R., R.M. Martha, and R. Evangelina. "Consumption of soft drinks with phosphoric acid as a risk factor for the development of hypocalcemia in postmenopausal women." *Journal of Clinical Epidemiology* Oct. 1999: 1007-1010.

Fisher, B., et al. "Tamoxifen for Prevention of Breast Cancer: Report of the National Surgical Adjuvant Breast and Bowel Project P-1 Study." *Journal of the National Cancer Institute,* 16 Sept. 1998: 572-578, 1371-1388.

Friedman, G.D., and A.L. Klatsky. "Is Alcohol Good for Your Health?" *New England Journal of Medicine* 16 Dec. 1993: 1882-1883.

Gartside, P.S., P. Wang, and C.J. Glueck. "Prospective assessment of coronary heart disease risk factors: The NHANES I Epidemiologic Follow-up Study (HNEFS) 16 follow up." *Journal of the American College of Nutrition.* 1999; 17: 263-269.

Gellar, A. "Common Addictions." *Clinical Symposia.* Ciba-Geigy Corporation. 1996.

Grossman, E., and F.H. Messerli. "Diabetic and Hypertensive Heart Disease." *Annals of Internal Medicine* 15 Aug. 1996: 304-310.

Harris, J.R., M.E. Lipman, M. Morrow, and S. Helman. Diseases of the Breast. Philadelphia: Lippencott and Raven. 1996.

Heaney, R.P. "Calcium — answers for lifelong health." Supplement to OBG Management. Dec. 1998.

Heaney, R.P. "Pathophysiology of Osteoporosis." *Endocrinology and Metabolism Clinics of North America* 27 June 1998: 255-265.

Henningfield, J.D., and R.M. Keenan. "The Anatomy of Nicotine Addiction." *Health Values* March/April 1993: 12-19.

Hutchings, O., et al. "Effect of early American results on patients in a Tamoxifen prevention trial." *Lancet* 10 Oct. 1998: 1222.

Joint National Committee. The Fifth Report of the Joint National Committee on Detection, Evaluation, and Treatment of High Blood Pressure. Bethesda (MD): National Institutes of Health, National Heart, Lung, and Blood Institute; 1993. NIH publication No. 93-1008.

Kannel, W.B., and R.B. D'Agostino, J.L. Cobb. "Effects of Weight on Cardiovascular Disease." *American Journal of Clinical Nutrition* March 1996: 419S-422S.

Kenney, W.L., et al. *American College of Sports Medicine Guidelines for Exercise Testing and Prescription*. 5th ed. Media, Pa.: Williams & Wilkins, 1995.

McCarron, D.A., and M.E. Reusser. "Body Weight and Blood Pressure Regulation." *American Journal of Clinical Nutrition* Mar. 1996: 423S-425S.

The Medical Letter. "Raloxifene for postmenopausal osteoporosis." Vol. 40 (Issue 1022), 13 March 1998.

Meeker, M.H., and J.C. Rothrock. *Alexander's Care of the Patient in Surgery*, 10th ed. St. Louis: Mosby, 1995.

Moline, M.L. "Pharmacologic strategies for managing premenstrual syndrome." *Clinical Pharmacokinetics*. 1993; 12: 181-196.

National Cancer Institute on breast cancer at http://www.nci.nih.gov accessed March 1999.

National Institutes of Health Consensus Development Conference Statement on Osteoporosis at http://www.osteo.org accessed March 1999.

Peterson, J.A., and C.X. Bryant. *The Fitness Handbook; 2nd ed.* St. Louis: Wellness Bookshelf, 1995.

Postgraduate Obstetrics and Gynecology. Management of Atypical and Low-grade Squamous Intraepithelial Pap Smears. March 1998. Volume 18. Number 6.

Prestwood, K.M., and A.M. Kenny. "Osteoporosis: pathogenesis, diagnosis, and treatment in older adults." *Clinics in Geriatric Medicine. 14 Aug. 1998: 577-599.*

Ryan, T.J., and J.L. Anderson, E.M. Autman, et al. "ACC/AHA Guidelines for the Management of Patients with Acute Myocardial Infarction: A Report of the American College of Cardiology/American Heart Association Task Force on Practice Guidelines (Committee on Management of Acute Myocardial Infarction)." *Journal of the American College of Cardiology* 1 Nov. 1996: 1328-1428.

St. Jeor, S.T., and K.D. Brownell, R.L. Atkinson, C. Bouchard, *et al.* "Obesity Workshop III." *Circulation 1996*: 1391-1396.
Scheiber, L.B., and L. Torregrosa. "Early intervention for postmenopausal osteoporosis." *Journal of Musculoskeletal Medicine* March 1999: 146-157, 276-285.
Schlant, R.C., and R.W. Alexander. *The Heart, 8th ed.* New York: McGraw-Hill, 1994.
Spense, A., and M. Elliot. Human Anatomy and Physiology, 3rd Ed. California: Benjamin/Cummings Publishing Company, Inc., 1987.
Speroff, L., R. Glass, and N. Kase. Clinical Gynecologic Endocrinology and Infertility, 5th Ed. Williams and Wilkins, 1994.
U.S. Department of Health and Human Services, NIH, NIA. "Osteoporosis: The Silent Bone Thinner." 1996.
United States Surgeon General. Department of Health and Human Services. *The Health Consequences of Smoking. Nicotine Addiction.* Washington, D.C.: U.S. Department of Health and Human Services, 1988.
United States Surgeon General on his priorities at http://www.osophs.dhhs.gov/myjob/priorities.htm accessed November 1999.
Wayne State University School of Medicine. "Vulvovaginal Candidiasis: A Contemporary Approach to Recognition and Management." Fall 1997.
Zelasko, C.J. "Exercise for Weight Loss: What Are the Facts?" *Journal of the American Dietetic Association* Dec. 1995: 973-1031.

For additional copies of
Women's Health Under 40: What You Should Know™,
contact your local bookseller
or call: (800) 289-0963.

For institutional quantities, call Joanne Widmer
at (800) 666-0963 ext. 262.

Other titles in the series *Your Health: What You Should Know™*:

Heart Disease: What You Should Know™

Congestive Heart Failure: What You Should Know™

Diabetes: What You Should Know™

High Cholesterol: What You Should Know™

Women's Health Over 40: What You Should Know™